From the publishers of the *Tarascon Pocket Pharmacopoeia*®

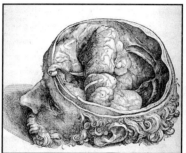

Courtesy of U.S. Library of Medicine

Melanie G. Hayden Gephart, MD, MAS

Department of Neurosurgery
Stanford University Hospital and Clinics
Stanford, CA

JONES & BARTLETT
L E A R N I N G

World Headquarters
Jones & Bartlett Learning
5 Wall Street
Burlington, MA 01803
978-443-5000
info@jblearning.com
www.jblearning.com

Jones & Bartlett Learning books and products are available through most bookstores and online booksellers. To contact Jones & Bartlett Learning directly, call 800-832-0034, fax 978-443-8000, or visit our website, www.jblearning.com.

Substantial discounts on bulk quantities of Jones & Bartlett Learning publications are available to corporations, professional associations, and other qualified organizations. For details and specific discount information, contact the special sales department at Jones & Bartlett Learning via the above contact information or send an email to specialsales@jblearning.com.

Production Credits
Sr. Acquisition Editor: Nancy Anastasi Duffy
Production Editor: Dan Stone
Digital Marketing Manager: Jennifer Sharp
Manufacturing and Inventory Control Supervisor: Amy Bacus
Composition: Newgen
Printing and Binding: Cenveo
Cover Printing: Cenveo
Cover Design: Kristin E. Parker
Cover Image: Courtesy of U.S. National Library of Medicine

ISBN 13: 978-0-7637-1554-3

6048

Printed in the United States of America
17 16 15 14 13 10 9 8 7 6 5 4 3 2 1

Dedicated to my family, colleagues, teachers, and patients.

I am eternally grateful.

Melanie

NOTE: To address the critical lack of trained neurosurgeons in developing countries, 100% of all proceeds of this book will be donated to the Foundation for International Education in Neurological Surgery (FIENS).

Tarascon Neurosurgery Pocketbook

Table of Contents

List of Contributors

EDITOR-IN-CHIEF

Melanie G. Hayden Gephart, MD, MAS
Neurosurgery Resident
Stanford University School of Medicine

CO-EDITOR
Gary K. Steinberg, MD, PhD
Chair of Neurosurgery
Lacroute-Hearst Professor of Neurosurgery and the Neurosciences
Department Neurosurgery
Stanford University School of Medicine

SECTION EDITORS
Michael SB Edwards, MD
Chair of Pediatric Neurosurgery, Professor of Neurosurgery
Lucile Packard Children's Hospital
Stanford University School of Medicine

Griffith Harsh, MD
Professor of Neurosurgery
Stanford University School of Medicine

Yuen So, MD, PhD
Professor of Neurology
Stanford University School of Medicine

CHAPTER EDITORS
Nancy Fischbein, MD
Associate Professor of Radiology
Stanford University School of Medicine

Raphael Guzman, MD
Lucile Packard Children's Hospital
Stanford University School of Medicine

Marco Lee, MD, PhD
Associate Professor of Neurosurgery
Stanford University School of Medicine

Jon Park, MD
Assistant Professor of Neurosurgery
Stanford University School of Medicine

Jeanette Phelps, PharmD
Pharmacist

Lawrence Shuer, MD
Professor of Neurosurgery
Stanford University School of Medicine

Hannes Vogel, MD
Associate Chair for Neuropathology, Professor of Pathology
Stanford University School of Medicine

CONTRIBUTORS

Scott Berta, MD
Neurosurgery Fellow
Stanford University School of Medicine

Kevin Chao, MD
Neurosurgery Resident
Stanford University School of Medicine

Jason Davies, MD
Neurosurgery Resident
Stanford University School of Medicine

Marie Gonella, MD
Neurology Resident
Stanford University School of Medicine

Lewis Hou, MD
Neurosurgery Resident
Stanford University School of Medicine

Maziar Kalani, BS
Medical Student
Stanford University School of Medicine

Paul Kalanithi, MD
Neurosurgery Resident
Stanford University School of Medicine

Gregory Kapinos, MD, MS
Assistant Professor of Neurosurgery
Hofstra North Shore-LIJ School of Medicine

Nandan Lad, MD, PhD
Neurosurgery Resident
Stanford University School of Medicine

Gordon Li, MD
Assistant Professor
Department of Neurosurgery
Stanford University School of Medicine

Robert Lober, MD
Neurosurgery Resident
Stanford University School of Medicine

David McCall, MD
Orthopedics Resident
Stanford University School of Medicine

Viet Nguyen, MD
Clinical Assistant Professor in Neurology
Stanford University School of Medicine

Gordon Sakamoto, MD
Neurosurgery Resident
Stanford University Hospital and Clinics

Keith Van Haren, MD
Neurology Resident
Stanford University School of Medicine

Anthony Wang, MD
Neurosurgery Resident
University of Michigan

FIGURE DESIGN
Andrew Phelps, MD
Assistant Professor of Clinical Radiology
University of California at San Francisco

I. NEUROLOGY

Griffith Harsh, MD
Michael SB Edwards, MD
Yuen So, MD, PhD

CHAPTER 1 ■ STROKE[1,2]

Melanie G. Hayden Gephart, MD, MAS
Anthony Wang, MD

Pathophysiology: Alteration in the blood supply to the brain → decreased oxygen delivery → neuronal cell death

- Causes of hypoxia include[3]: Low blood oxygen content (carbon monoxide poisoning, drowning, respiratory arrest), ischemia, or decreased tissue oxygen utilization (cyanide toxicity)
- Stroke classically defined by either vessel rupture (hemorrhagic) or vessel occlusion (ischemic)

Risk factors[4]: Age, transient ischemic attack (TIA), smoking (2-fold), atrial fibrillation (5-fold), hypertension (> 120/80), race (increased in African American), hypercholesterolemia

Hemorrhagic stroke: Cerebral arteries prone to hemorrhage because they have no elastic laminae (Charcot-Bouchard microaneurysm in hypertension)

- Basal ganglia, pons, thalamus are affected more frequently because perforators branch directly from high pressure arteries
- Additional causes include: Cerebrovascular malformation, vasculitis, amyloidosis, drug use (e.g., cocaine or methamphetamine), collagen/vascular disorders, area of prior ischemic stroke, anticoagulation, neoplasia

Ischemic stroke:

- Cortex layers particularly sensitive to hypoxia: Hippocampus (CA1, CA4), cortex (watershed, parietal-occipital layers[2,3,5]), basal ganglia (caudate, putamen), cerebellum (Purkinje's cells), thalamus
- Cortex layers particularly resistant to hypoxia: hippocampus CA2, cortex (Ufibers, extreme and external capsules)
- Additional causes include: arterial dissection (vertebral, carotid, aortic), embolic (e.g., cardiac, septic, cholesterol), antiphospholipid antibody syndrome, thrombolytic thrombocytopenic purpura, vasculitis, venous sinus thrombosis

Incidence[4]: 700,000 strokes/year

- Third leading cause of death in the United States
- In adults > 55 years old, risk is 1:6
- 87% of strokes are ischemic
- Prevalence of "silent" strokes 11–40% at > 55 years of age

Symptoms/Signs: See Tables 1-1 and 1-2

Assessment: ABCs, GCS

- Start O_2, IV, EKG, cardiac enzymes
- Evaluate 3-hour window for IV tPA
- Determine NIH stroke scale (see Appendix 1)

Table 1-1 Stroke Signs and Symptoms by Location

Ischemic Stroke		
Vascular territory	*Vessel*	*Possible localizing signs*
Anterior	ICA, MCA, ACA	Left: Aphasia, right-sided weakness Right: Left hemi-neglect, left-sided weakness, denial of deficit
Posterior	PCA	Left: Right hemianopsia, alexia without agraphia Right: Left hemianopsia
Vertebrobasilar	Vertebral, basilar	Cranial nerve palsies, vertigo, quadriparesis, nystagmus, ataxia, coma
Lacunar motor	Perforators to pons or internal capsule	Pure hemiparesis
Lacunar sensory	Perforators to thalamus or posterior limb of internal capsule	Pure hemisensory deficits

Hemorrhagic Stroke	
Location	*Possible localizing signs*
Putamen/internal capsule	Contralateral hemiparesis and sensory loss, contralateral conjugate gaze paresis (look toward lesion)
Thalamus	Contralateral sensory loss, upgaze paralysis, somnolence, aphasia or neglect, pupil constriction, ipsilateral conjugate gaze paresis (look away from lesion)
Lobar	Confusion, aphasia, neglect, hemianopsia, contralateral conjugate gaze paresis
Caudate	Contralateral hemiplegia, agitation, memory deficit, ipsilateral Horner's syndrome
Cerebellum	Nystagmus, vertigo, ataxia, ipsilateral pupil constriction
Pons	Quadriparesis, coma, pupil constriction, ocular bobbing, horizontal gaze palsy, cranial nerve deficits

- Labs: CBC, chemistry, coags, type and screen, glucose, tox screen
- Imaging: CT head to rule out hemorrhage, consider CT-Angio (to include cervical spine if history of trauma to rule out carotid dissection), MRI stroke protocol (See Table 1-2); echocardiogram, carotid duplex U/S

Treatment: Permissive hypertension if ischemic to 220/120 (185/110 for tPA), mean arterial pressure < 90 if hemorrhagic

- Avoid hypotonic fluids
- Avoid hyperglycemia
- Maintain normothermia

Table 1-2 Hematomal Appearance on the MRI

Stage	Time from Stroke	T1	T2
Hyperacute	4–6 hours	Isointense	Hyperintense
Acute	7–72 hours	Isointense	Hypointense
Early subacute	4–7 days	Hyperintense	Hypointense
Late subacute	1–4 weeks	Hyperintense	Hyperintense
Early chronic	weeks to months	Hyperintense	Hyperintense
Late chronic	months to years	Hypointense	Hypointense

Table 1-3 Criteria for Stroke Treatment with tPA[1]

Inclusion	Contraindications
• Clinical diagnosis of stroke with significant, nonresolving deficit • Age > 18 years • < 3 hours from last known to be neurologically intact • ICU level of care available • Noncontrast head CT without evidence of hemorrhage	History: • history of CNS hemorrhage, aneurysm, or AVM • seizure at stroke onset • ongoing acute myocardial infarction • recent arterial puncture at noncompressible site • no lumbar puncture within 7 days • major surgery or serious trauma within 14 days • GI/GU bleed within 21 days • lactation or pregnancy within last 30 days • head trauma/bleed/surgery or stroke within 3 months Vitals: • SBP > 185, DBP > 110 Laboratory analysis: • platelets < 100,000 • treated with heparin within 48 hours • INR > 1.7 • blood glucose < 50 or > 400

- Manage intracranial hypertension (hyperventilation, diuresis, hemicraniectomy)
- Possible treatment, depending upon etiology: tPA (see Table 1-3), preventative (aspirin, statin, anti-hypertensives), carotid endarterectomy
- If clinical status deteriorates, stop tPA infusion and order STAT head CT and appropriate labs
- If hemorrhage present, correct thrombolysis with cryoprecipitate, FFP, and platelets
- Consult neurosurgery when appropriate for consideration of surgical decompression or clot evacuation

Outcome: Associated with significant morbidity, depending upon extent and location of stroke

- Mean lifetime cost of $140,000[4]
- Cost of stroke in 2007 was 62.7 billion dollars
- Complications of tPA Treatment: 6% overall rate of symptomatic intracerebral hemorrhage

VENOUS INFARCT AKA CEREBRAL VENOUS SINUS THROMBOSIS[6]

Occlusion of a venous sinus or cortical vein (thrombus or external compression)

Etiology: Hypercoagulable state (pregnancy, hormonal replacement or birth control pills, Factor V Leiden mutation, antiphospholipid antibody syndrome, activated protein C resistance, elevated factor VIII, malignancy, protein C and protein S deficiency, homocystinuria, trauma, sticky platelet syndrome), dehydration, tumor, infection

Imaging: MRI/MRV (venogram)

- Distribution unusual for arterial infarct (deep white matter)
- High risk for hemorrhagic conversion

AMYLOID ANGIOPATHY[7,8,9]

Pathophysiology: Deposition of beta-amyloid in the media and adventitia of small and mid-sized arteries

- Morphologic hallmarks of Alzheimer's disease (AD)
- Primary amyloid (secondary in DM, beta microglobulin)

Incidence[10]: Seen in up to 36% of autopsy specimens

- Frequently presents in the elderly as dementia, lobar intraparencymal hemorrhage (15% of ICH) in normotension (rostral parietal area, corticomedullary junction)
- Most sporadic, occasional familial

Treatment: Supportive

- Surgery may be considered in patients with intermediate-sized hematomas (20–60 mL) who progressively deteriorate in their level of consciousness

Outcome: Recurrence rate of 38% with mortality rate of 44%

STROKE SYNDROMES[4,11]

ANTON SYNDROME

- Bilateral occipital lobe strokes
- Bilateral PCA or top of the basilar syndrome
- Visual deficit without recognition of blindness (visual agnosia)

BALINT SYNDROME

- Bilateral posterior cerebral artery (parietal-occipital)
- Loss of voluntary but not reflexive eye movements
- Optic ataxia
- Asimultagnosia

CLAUDE'S (DORSAL MIDBRAIN) SYNDROME

- Ipsilateral CNIII palsy with contralateral ataxia

DEJERINE (MEDIAL MEDULLARY) SYNDROME

- Basilar artery, vertebral artery, anterior spinal artery
- Contralateral spastic weakness (pyramidal tract) that spares face
- Loss of vibration/position sense (medial lemniscus)
- Ipsilateral tongue weakness (CN XII nucleus)

DEJERINE-ROUSSY SYNDROME

- PCA thalamic perforators
- Hemisensory loss
- Hemibody pain

FOVILLE'S (INFERIOR MEDIAL PONTINE) SYNDROME

- Basilar artery perforators
- Contralateral weakness (corticospinal)
- Facial weakness (CN VII nucleus)
- Lateral gaze deficit (CN VI nucleus)
- Decreased sensation/vibration sense (medial lemniscus)

GERSTMANN SYNDROME

- Dominant parietal lobe (MCA)
- Agraphia
- Acalculia
- Left-right confusion
- Finger agnosia
- Ideomotor apraxia

LOCKED-IN SYNDROME

- Basilar artery
- Paralysis of all movement except vertical gaze and eyelid opening (supranuclear ocular motor pathway preserved)
- Sensation and consciousness preserved (reticular formation spared)

MARIE-FOIX (LATERAL INFERIOR PONTINE) SYNDROME

- AICA occlusion
- Ipsilateral ataxia (cerebellar tract)
- Nausea, vertigo, decreased hearing (vestibular nucleus)
- Contralateral hemiparesis (corticospinal tract)

- Ipsilateral facial weakness (facial nucleus)
- Ipsilateral loss of facial sensation (spinal trigeminal nucleus)
- Contralateral hemihypesthesis (spinothalamic tract)

MILLARD-GUBLER (VENTRAL PONTINE) SYNDROME

- Basilar artery perforators
- Base of pons syndrome
- Contralateral weakness (corticospinal tract)
- Diplopia, strabismus, loss of extroversion (CN VI)
- Ipsilateral facial weakness (VII)

RAYMOND (VENTRAL PONTINE) SYNDROME

- Perforators of basilar artery
- Lateral gaze deficits (CN VI)
- Weakness (pyramidal tract)

TOP OF THE BASILAR SYNDROME

- Sudden onset of altered mental status
- Ophthalmoplegia, papillary, and visual field (homonymous hemianopsia) abnormalities
- Generally embolic or postangio stent complication

WALLENBERG (LATERAL MEDULLARY) SYNDROME

- Most commonly from verterbral artery occlusion or dissection, classically a posterior inferior cerebellar artery occlusion
- Facial pain and sensory loss (trigeminal nucleus)
- Ataxia (restiform body and peduncle of cerebellum)
- Nystagmus, nausea, vomiting, vertigo (vestibular nucleus)
- Hoarseness, dysphagia, dysarthria, loss of gag (nucleus ambiguus, glossopharyngeal nucleus or exiting intra-axial fibers → ipsilateral lower motor neuron paralysis of the larynx and soft palate)
- Loss of taste (solitary nucleus)
- Ipsilateral Horner's syndrome (sympathetics)
- Contralateral hemisensory loss of pain and temperature (spinothalamic tract), ipsilateral numbness (cuneate/gracile nuclei)
- Hiccups (reticulophrenic)

WEBER SYNDROME

- PCA midbrain perforators leading to ventral midbrain infarct
- Contralateral weakness (corticospinal tract)
- Lateral gaze deficits and ipsilateral pupillary dilation (CN3)
- Contralateral corticobulbar dysfunction

CHAPTER 2 ■ SEIZURES[1-12]

Gregory Kapinos, MD, MS
Keith Van Haren, MD

TEMPORAL LOBE EPILEPSY

Epidemiology: Most common epilepsy syndrome of adults (70% of patients with complex partial seizures)

- Present in childhood/adolescence
- Predisposition with febrile seizures of infancy

Etiology: May be mesial temporal sclerosis (cause or consequence)

Seizure type: Simple partial or complex partial, from mesial temporal lobe (hippocampus, amygdala, parahippocampal gyrus → auras, visceral sensations, automatisms, postictal confusion, may have secondary generalization)

Treatment: Carbamazepine may prevent generalization

- If refractory may require temporal lobectomy

MEDICAL TREATMENT OF SEIZURES (TABLE 2.1)

AED SELECTION[1,4]

■ **Generalized Onset**
1st line: Carbamazepine, Lamotrigine, Oxcarbazepine, Phenobarbital, Phenytoin, Topiramate, Valproate
- *2nd line* Levetiracetam, Primidone, Zonisamide

■ **Partial onset**
1st line: Carbamazepine*, Phenytoin*, Valproate*, Gabapentin, Lamotrigine, Oxcarbazepine, Phenobarbital, Topiramate, Vigabatrin
- *2nd line* Levetiracetam, Pregabalin, Primidone, Tiagabine, Zonisamide

*most commonly used 1st line drugs because of higher level of evidence

SURGICAL TREATMENT OF MEDICALLY REFRACTORY SEIZURES

■ **Focal Lesionectomy**
Resection of focal epileptic origin from noneloquent area of the brain
- Lesion location diagnosed by MRI, PET, continuous EEG monitoring with scalp or subdural electrodes

Table 2-1 Antiepileptic Drug Table

Drug	Start Dose	Titration	Maintain	Serum Levels	Clearance/Half-life	Mechanism	Unique SEs
Carbamazepine Tegretol – TID Teg XR – BID Carbatrol – BID	200 mg BID 200 mg BID	200 mg/day qwk	200–400 mg TID 400–600 mg BID	• 4–12 mcg/mL • 70% protein bound	• hepatic cytochrome P-450 (CYP) • 12–17 hrs	• voltage-dep Na channels	• CYP450 • hyponatremia • neurotoxicity • leukopenia, aplastic anemia • SJS/TEN • hepatitis **HLA-B 1502 testing in Asian pts predicts rash
Ethosuximide Zarontin	250 mg BID	250 mg q4d	500 mg BID	40–100 mcg/mL	• hepatic • 30–60 hrs	• T-type Ca current in thalamus	• insomnia • pancytopenia • hyperactivity
Felbamate Felbatol	400 mg TID	600 mg/day q2 wk	1200 mg TID		• CYP450 • 24 hrs	• NMDAR antagonist • GABA	• aplastic anemia • hepatotoxicity • anorexia
Gabapentin Neurontin	300 mg qd	variable	300–1600 mg TID		• renal • 4–6 hrs	• voltage dep Ca • inc I(H) current CA1 hippocampus • GABA(B) → dec glutamate	• sedation • weight gain

Lamotrigine *Lamictal*	1st 2 wks—50 mg qd; 2nd 2 wks—50 mg BID	25–50 mg qwk (100 mg/day q1–2 wks)	150–250 mg BID (monotherapy)	1.5–1C mcg/mL	• liver glucuronidation • renal excretion • 10–60 hrs	• Na channels blocking	• rash/SJS/TEN • angioedema • multiorgan failure/DIC • somnolence • drug interaction • myoclonus
Levetiracetam *Keppra*	500 mg BID	500 mg q2 wks	1000 mg BID		• renal • 6–12 hrs	• binds SV2A and inhibits presynaptic Ca2+ channels	• URI • aggression • depression
Oxcarbazepine *Trileptal*	150–300 mg BID	300 mg/d every 3 days	600 mg BID		• hepatic • 8–10 hrs	• voltage-dep Na channels	• hypothyroid • SJS/TEN/rash • induces CYP450 • angioedema • hyponatremia
Phenobarbital	100–300 mg/d divided qd TID	none	300 mg/d divided TID	15–40 mcg/rL	• hepatic • 24–100 hrs	• GABA(A) R → inc duration of Cl channel opening	• lethargy • impaired cognition • fetal malformation

(Continued)

Table 2-1 Antiepileptic Drug Table (Continued)

Drug	Start dose	Titration	Maintain	Serum Levels	Clearance/Half-life	Mechanism	Unique SEs
Phenytoin *Dilantin* **Fosphenytoin** *Cerebyx*	400 mg initial IV load for status epilepticus: 15–20 mg/kg	300 mg in 2 hrs & 4 hrs	200–500 mg/d div qd (extended release) to TID (immediate release)	• 10–20 mcg/mL • Free level: 1–2 mcg/mL	• Hepatic amine oxidase • 7–40 hrs	• voltage-dep Na channels • synaptic trans • Ca-calmodulin phosphorylation	• gingival hypertrophy • osteomalacia • fetal malformation • hirsutism • rash/SJS/TEN • lymphadenopathy
Pregabalin *Lyrica*	75 mg BID	75 mg qwk	150–300 mg BID		• renal • 6 hrs	• voltage-gated Ca • glutamate, norepi, subst P	• euphoria • myoclonus • weight gain
Tiagabine *Gabitril*	2 mg BID	4–8 mg/d qwk	32–56 mg/d div BID to QID		• hepatic • 4–8 hrs	• Inhibits GABA reuptake	• dizziness • fatigue, weakness • rash • seizures
Topiramate *Topamax*	25 mg BID	Wk 2: 50 mg BID; Wk 3: 75 mg BID; Wk 4: 100 mg BID; Wk 5: 150 mg BID	100–200 mg BID		• renal • 20 hrs	• GABA (A) Rs • NMDAR antagonist • weak CA inhi	• cognitive difficulties • weight loss • mood • somnolence • metabolic acidosis • nephrolithiasis

Valproate Depakote Depakene Depakote ER	10–15 mg/kg/d divided BID–TID 10–15 mg/kg qd	5–10 mg/kg qwk	60 mg/kg/d 60 mg/kg/d	• 50–150 mcg/mL • light protein bound	• hepatic oxidation, conjugation • 9–12 hrs	• voltage-dep Na channels • increases GABA • T-type Ca	• weight gain • insulin resist • thrombocytopenia • hepatotoxicity • fetal malformation • pancreatitis • hyperammonanemia
Vigabatrin not available in the US	40 mg/kg/d div BID	30–40 mg/kg qwk	40–100 mg/kg/d div BID		• renal • 6–8 hrs	• Irreversible GABA-transaminase inhibitor	• concentric visual field loss • depression • weight gain
Zonisamide Zonegran	100 mg qd	100 mg/d q2wks	200–400 mg qd		• hepatic/renal • 60 hrs	• Sulfonamide derivative • Voltage dep Na and T-type Ca channels • CA inhibitor	• renal stones • anorexia • rash/SJS • agranulcytosis

BID = two times per day; TID = three times per day; QID = four times per day; QD = once per day

▓ Temporal Lobectomy
Mesial temporal sclerosis
- Complications: Superior quadrantanopia, third nerve palsy, aphasia (dominant), stroke, hemorrhage, paralysis

▓ Corpus Callosotomy
Division of anterior two thirds of the corpus callosum
- To limit secondary generalization (atonic seizures, generalized tonic-clonic)
- Complication: Left/right dissociation, hemorrhage, retraction or vaccine injury

▓ Vagal Nerve Stimulator
Intermittent electrical stimulation of vagus nerve indicated for treatment of medically refractory seizures → decreased seizure frequency/duration and enabling decrease of medication
- Side effects: Cough, hoarseness, paresthesia, dyspnea
- Performed only on the left side so that cardiac innervation by the vagus is unaffected

CHAPTER 3 ■ COMMUNICATION DISORDERS[1,2]

Melanie G. Hayden Gephart, MD, MAS

ANATOMY OF LANGUAGE

95% of individuals' language center is in the left, dominant hemisphere

- A small percentage of left-handed individuals have bilateral innervation
- Important to distinguish sensory (visual, auditory) from the motor ability to formulate or perceive language

BROCA'S AREA

Location: Inferior frontal gyrus of dominant hemisphere, anterior to motor cortex for mouth/tongue, middle cerebral artery territory

Function: Controls expressive language (ability to coordinate muscle movements and produce the complex sounds and intonations associated with language)

WERNICKE'S AREA

Location: Superior temporal gyrus, auditory association cortex

Function: Language comprehension (speech, writing, signs, etc.)

ARCUATE FASCICULUS: White matter tract connecting Broca's and Wernicke's areas

ANGULAR GYRUS

Posterior temporal-parietal junction

- At the end of the superior temporal sulcus and continuous with the middle temporal gyrus
- Involved in visual function and in the dominant hemisphere (generally left sided), functions in language, specifically comprehension of writing

APHASIA

BROCA'S APHASIA (EXPRESSIVE OR NONFLUENT)

Lesion: Broca's area

Symptoms/Signs: Difficulty with language production, however, comprehension is intact

- Agrammatism, anomia
- Repetition impaired

- Patient acutely aware of deficits
- Due to location near motor cortex, may also involve contralateral motor weakness (arm > leg)

WERNICKE'S APHASIA (RECEPTIVE OR FLUENT)

Lesion: Wernicke's area

Symptoms/Signs: Ease with production of speech, however, content is classically nonsensical

- Neologisms, literal and verbal paraphasias, circumlocutory
- Difficulty with language comprehension, repetition, and following verbal commands
- Patient may be unaware of deficit

CONDUCTIVE APHASIA

Lesion: Injury of the arcuate fasciculus

Symptoms/Signs: Results in difficulties with repetition as the connection between Broca's and Wernicke's areas has been disrupted

- Anomia

GLOBAL APHASIA

Lesion: Involvement of Broca's, Wernicke's, and the arcuate fasciculus

- Usually secondary to large strokes of the middle cerebral artery of the dominant hemisphere

Symptoms/Signs: Leads to a dense expressive and receptive aphasia

PROGRESSIVE NONFLUENT APHASIA

Anatomy: Atrophy of frontal/temporal lobes (perisylvian)

Symptoms/Signs: Dementia with agrammatism, phonemic paraphasia, anomia

- Later may develop behavioral changes (variant of frontotemporal dementia)
- May progress to dysarthria/mutism

SEMANTIC APHASIA

Anatomy: Atrophy of anterior temporal lobe

Symptoms/Signs: Fluent

- No knowledge of word meaning
- Semantic paraphasias
- No memory deficits
- Prosopagnosia
- Alexia
- Later may develop behavioral changes (variant of frontotemporal dementia)

ADDITIONAL LANGUAGE DISORDERS

ANOMIA

Lesion: Can occur secondary to focal cortical lesion in the dominant hemisphere or global encephalopathy

Symptoms/Signs: Inability to name an object when presented

- May occur as part of a fluent aphasia
- Repetition and comprehension generally intact

Pure Word Deafness: Cannot understand spoken words, but can hear sounds and understands written language

- Results from temporal lobe lesion

ALEXIA

Lesion: Classically associated with lesions of the angular gyrus (posterior temporal-parietal)

Symptoms/Signs: Inability to read

- Can be with or without agraphia
- May be associated with aphasia

AGNOSIA

Lesion: Nondominant (usually right) temporal-parietal lobe

Symptoms/Signs: Inability to recognize and identify objects or persons

- Can be limited to one sensory modality (e.g., auditory, gustatory, olfactory, tactile, or visual)

Anosognosia: Denial of a physical deficit (e.g. hemiparalysis); when shown the paralyzed body part patient may deny that it is his or hers

- Usually associated with hemi-neglect

VERBAL APRAXIA

- Developmental or acquired
- Impairment involving planning, executing, and sequencing of speech

AGRAPHIA

- Inability to compose written language

DYSARTHRIA

Lesion: Disruption of speech mechanics, i.e., corticobulbar (cranial nerve nuclei or cranial nerves), cerebellar (coordination), or musculature of speech production

Symptoms/Signs: Decreased phonation, poor articulation, and changes in resonance/respiration

- Composition of speech is normal

CHAPTER 4 ■ NEURO-OPHTHALMOLOGY AND NEUROTOLOGY

Marie Gonella, MD

Melanie G Hayden Gephart, MD, MAS

NYSTAGMUS[1,2]

- In central vertigo, horizontal, rotary, or vertical nystagmus may be present and may be bidirectional
- In peripheral vertigo, nystagmus should be horizontal and unidirectional or rotary
- Direction is described by the direction of the fast phase
- Should fatigue (lessen) with repeated testing

Abducting: Intranuclear ophthalmoplegia (INO), pontine medial longitudinal fasciculus

Brun's: Pontomedullary junction

Convergence: Adducting nystagmus

- Pineal lesion
- Seen with Parinaud's syndrome

Dissociated: See INO (usually multiple sclerosis [MS])

Downbeat: Disruption between cerebellum and brainstem

- Posterior fossa lesion (cervicomedullary junction/foramen magnum; e.g., chiari, bilateral cerebellar lesions, cerebellar tumor), basilar invagination, metabolic, multiple sclerosis, spinocerebellar degeneration, bilateral MLF lesions, platybasia

Horizontal: Peripheral etiology

Ocular bobbing: From large, destructive lesion of the pons

Opsoclonus: Myoclonic triangle

- "Dancing eyes"; chaotic, unrelenting saccadic movements in all directions
- Associated with viral infection (encephalitis) or tumors (commonly pediatric)

Optokinetic: Physiologic

- Brought out by black lines on white background
- Impaired in parietal lesions (not occipital)

Periodic alternating, square wave jerks: Conjugate, horizontal

- Cerebellum

Retractorius: Co-contraction of all extraocular muscles

- Midbrain tegmentum lesion (e.g., pineal tumor, stroke)

Rotary: Jerk (fast and slow phase) and pendular (equal velocity oscillations)

- Disruption of semicircular canals, brain stem/cerebellum lesion
- May be associated with vision loss
- Lateral medullary syndrome (fast away from lesion side)
- Accentuated on lateral gaze
- Vestibular system dysfunction (see with horizontal/vertical nystagmus)

Seesaw: Intorting eye up, extorting eye down

- Diencephalic or parasellar lesion, chiasmal compression

Spasmus mutans: Nystagmus, head nodding torticollis

- Infants

Upbeat: Medulla

PAPILLEDEMA

Secondary to axoplasmic stasis
- Generally takes 24–48 hours to develop (not before 6 hours)
- Causes include pseudotumor cerebri, mass lesion, multiple sclerosis (acute optic neuritis and pale disks as a result of past optic neuritis); patient may be obtunded (increased intracranial pressure) and have nausea and vomiting

■ DDx of Unilateral Papilledema[2]
Tumor (orbital, meningioma, optic glioma), inflammatory, Foster Kennedy syndrome, demyelination

FOSTER KENNEDY SYNDROME[3]
Direct pressure on the optic nerve from a mass lesion (e.g., tumor) → ipsilateral anosmia, ipsilateral scotoma with optic atrophy (direct pressure on optic nerve → visual loss), contralateral papilledema (→ enlarged blind spot) secondary to increased intracranial pressure
- May have visual loss in the atrophic eye

PSEUDO-FOSTER KENNEDY SYNDROME[4]
More common
- Remote ischemia or demyelination in one eye leading to atrophy (chronic visual loss) and new ischemia or demyelination in the second eye (new visual loss)

CONJUGATE GAZE[5]

1. Super nuclear gaze center (SNGC) located in the frontal lobe receives voluntary input from bilateral hemispheres, cerebellum, vestibular nuclei, neck, and initiates saccadic eye movement to the contralateral side
   • SNGC lesion causes deviation to the affected side

2. SNGC corticobulbar fibers travel through the genu of the internal capsule and synapse with the ipsilateral pontine gaze center (PGC) located at the parapontine reticular formation (PPRF aka horizontal gaze center)
   • PGC directs eye movement to the ipsilateral side
   • Caudal PPRF stimulation leads to conjugate, ipsilateral horizontal eye deviation, whereas rostral PPRF stimulation leads to vertical eye movement

3. Fibers from PGC synapse with the ipsilateral CNVI (abducens) nucleus and crosses via medial longitudinal fasciculus (MLF) to synapse with the contralateral CN III nucleus (medial rectus)
   • MLF contains fibers from interstitial nucleus of Cajal, medial vestibular nucleus, pontine reticular formation, superior colliculus
   • Inhibitory signals travel to the opposing medial rectus
   • Lesion of PGC causes eye deviation to the side opposite the lesion
   • Lesion at MLF causes loss of adduction of the ipsilateral eye and nystagmus of the contralateral eye on abduction

HORIZONTAL GAZE PALSY

Commonly from injury to the horizontal gaze center or CNVI nucleus → loss of horizontal gaze *ipsilateral* to the lesion
   • Range in severity from complete (nonresponsive to voluntary or vestibular control) to nystagmus with stimulation
   • Usually secondary to stroke

VERTICAL GAZE PALSY

MLF fibers and nucleus, cranial nerve nuclei, interstitial nucleus of Cajal, superior colliculus → rostral interstitial nucleus of the MLF
   • Causes: Tumors (e.g., midbrain glioma, pineal tumor), stroke (midbrain pretectum), increased ICP (Parinaud's syndrome aka dorsal midbrain syndrome), progressive supranuclear palsy (impaired downward gaze with preservation of upward gaze)

■ Parinaud's Syndrome[6]

Vertical gaze palsy, lid retraction (Collier's sign), "setting-sun" sign (downward gaze preference), light near dissociation, convergence retraction nystagmus

SUPRANUCLEAR GAZE PALSY

   • SNGC (frontal lobe) normally directs conjugate deviation of the eyes to the opposite side

- Presents with ipsilateral conjugate eye deviation despite preservation of brainstem reflexive conjugate eye movement

PONTINE GAZE PALSY

Limits ipsilateral gaze (abducens nucleus), causing eye deviation away from the lesion (toward the hemiparesis)
- Lesion of the pontine horizontal gaze center
- May be associated with hemiparesis

INTERNUCLEAR OPHTHALMOPLEGIA (INO)

(Figure 4.1): Lesion of the MLF leads to lateral gaze palsy
- Ipsilateral eye cannot adduct when looking to contralateral side
- Nystagmus in the adducting eye contralateral to the medial longitudinal fasciculus lesion
- *Can still ADduct on convergence* (differentiates this from a cranial nerve palsy where the eye cannot ADduct even when attempting to converge)

ONE-AND-A-HALF SYNDROME[7]

(Figure 4.2): Conjugate horizontal gaze palsy in one direction (lesion of the lateral gaze center/PPRF or abducens nucleus) in addition to an internuclear ophthalmoplegia in the other (lesion of the ipsilateral MLF → failure of adduction of ipsilateral eye)
- Prevents the eye ipsilateral to the PPRF from moving horizontally in either direction while the contralateral eye is only able to ABduct
- Most commonly caused by multiple sclerosis

CN III (OCULOMOTOR NERVE) PALSY

Affected side has ptosis, dilated pupil, ADducted and inferior gaze (unopposed CN IV and VI)

CN IV (TROCHLEAR NERVE) PALSY

Controls the superior oblique muscle (intorts, depresses, and ABducts the eye)

Symptoms: Vertical or torsinal diplopia

- Leads to head tilt away from the lesion to compensate (Bielschowsky's sign; in kids may be misdiagnosed as torticollis)
- Diplopia worsens when looking down (e.g., walking down stairs)

DDx: Trauma, congenital, iatrogenic, stroke, multiple sclerosis, tumor, thyroid, myasthenia, aneurysm

CN VI (ABDUCENS NERVE) PALSY[1]

(Figure 4.3): CN VI controls the lateral rectus muscle (ABducts the ipsilateral eye) has longest intracranial course, therefore, is more susceptible to traumatic shearing, stretching with tension on dura or increased intracranial pressure (ICP)

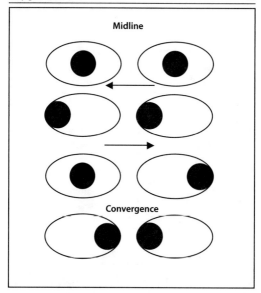

Figure 4-1 Internuclear Ophthalmoplegia (Right)

Symptoms: Binocular horizontal diplopia, ipsilateral esotropia in primary gaze

DDx: Multiple sclerosis (most common cause of isolated palsy), diabetes, temporal arteritis, increased ICP (hydrocephalus, pseudotumor, tumor), trauma, aneurysm, carotid-cavernous fistula, tumor, inflammation, intracranial hypotension (CSF leak, e.g., after lumbar puncture), skull-based fracture (e.g., clivus), mastoiditis (Gradenigo syndrome)

■ Gradenigo Syndrome

Otalgia (ophthalmic branch of trigeminal nerve), ipsilateral paralysis of abducens nerve, otitis media/mastoiditis (involving apex of petrous temporal bone)

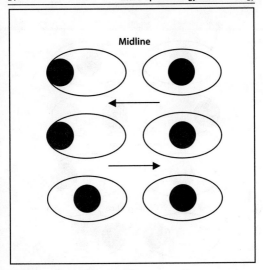

Figure 4-2 One-and-a-Half Syndrome

TOLOSA-HUNT SYNDROME[8]

Granuloma of superior orbital fissure; required for diagnosis
- Painful, unilateral ophthalmoplegia
- May extend into the cavernous sinus to involve any nerve there (generally lateral wall: CN III, V1, V2, VI)
- Pupil sparing
- Treat with high-dose steroids

FOIX SYNDROME

Syndrome of the superior orbital fissure (through which passes CN III, IV, V1, VI)

Symptoms: Ophthalmoplegia, corneal anesthesia, proptosis, pupillary dilation

DDx: Tumor, aneurysm, trauma (facial fracture)

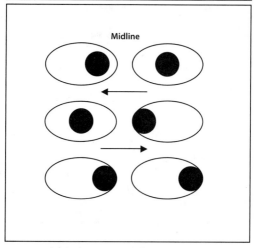

Figure 4-3 Abducens Nerve (CNVI) Palsy (Right)

PUPILLARY REFLEX AND ABERRATIONS IN PUPIL SIZE AND REACTIVITY[2,9]

PUPILLARY LIGHT REFLEX

CN II afferent, CN III efferent
- Unilateral light → retinal photoreceptors → optic nerve (CN II) → hemidecussation at the optic chiasm → optic tracts → exit optic tracts before the lateral geniculate body (LGN) → enter the brainstem in the brachium of the superior colliculus → synapse in pretectal olivary and sublentiform nuclei → cross in posterior commissure and ventral to the cerebral aqueduct to bilateral Edinger-Westphal nuclei → pupillary fibers travel with CN III (oculomotor) to ciliary ganglia → short ciliary nerve to iris sphincter, ciliary body → bilateral pupillary constriction

Pupillary sympathetic pathway: Hypothalamus to lateral horn cells of C8-T3 → superior cervical ganglion → iris

DIFFERENTIAL DIAGRAM OF PUPILLARY ABNORMALITIES

Amaurotic: Optic nerve lesion

- Equal sized pupils; normal direct, consensual, and near reflex

CN III compression: From interruption of more peripheral, circumferential parasympathetic fibers, leads to pupillary dilation

- Uncal herniation (accompanied by decreased level of consciousness), aneurysm, (CN III compression by posterior communicating artery aneurysm, classically involves the pupil)

Tonic (Adie's) pupil: Postganglionic parasympathetic interruption (ciliary ganglion)

- Women, 30–40s
- Loss of direct or consensual light reflex, light-near dissociation
- 0.125% pilocarpine in both eyes → constriction of affected pupil (denervation hypersensitivity) but not in normal pupil
- Reinnervation allows pupil to constrict
- May occur with pineal region tumors

CN III neuropathy: Controls superior rectus, medial rectus, inferior rectus, inferior oblique

- Lesion leads to inferiorly abducted eye with ptosis and pupillary dilation from DM (thought to be from ischemic vasculopathy as it spares the more peripheral parasympathetic fibers → pupil sparing CN III palsy), drugs (scopolamine, tropicamide, phenelyephrine)

Traumatic iridoplegia

Marcus-Gunn pupil (afferent pupillary defect): Consensual reflex stronger than direct—retina or optic nerve lesion, e.g., MS

Argyll Robertson pupil: Accommodates but doesn't react (light-near dissociation), tertiary syphilis, midbrain lesion

Pupil sparing oculomotor palsy: DM, atherosclerosis, temporal arteritis, chronic progressive ophthalmoplegia, myasthenia gravis

Pupil involving oculomotor palsy: Tumor (chordomas, mengioma), vascular (posterior communicating), uncal herniation, cavernous sinus lesion (also involves V1, V2, IV, VI—cavernous sinus syndrome)

Horner's syndrome: Interruption of sympathetics at a central, pre- or postganglionic location → miosis, anhydrosis, ptosis

- Differentiate pre- from postganglionic sympathetic denervation via administration of hydroxyamphetamine 1% (stimulates endogenous norepi release → pupillary dilation if preganglionic, no mydriasis if postganglionic)
- DDx includes cluster headache, cavernous sinus disease

Ross syndrome: Adie's tonic pupil (increased papillary diameter and sluggish constriction to light), excessive sweating, decreased deep tendon reflexes (especially Achilles), occasionally cardiovascular abnormalities

- Generally starts unilateral, then progresses to the other side
- Young women
- Caused by inflammation/damage to the cilliary and spinal ganglia

CORTICAL VISUAL ABNORMALITIES

BALINT'S SYNDROME

Visual inattention
- Cannot gaze to a specific point in visual field
- Extraocular movements intact
- Caused by bilateral parieto-occipital lesions

PROSOPAGNOSIA

Inability to identify familiar faces (e.g., of close friends or family); from a lesion of the right fusiform gyrus

ACHROMATOPSIA

Inability to recognize colors
- From occipitotemporal lesion

NEUROTOLOGY

VERTIGO

Important to distinguish from syncope/near syncope or disequilibrium and clarify "dizziness"

- Vertigo can be peripheral or central in origin

Peripheral causes: Include benign positional vertigo (BPV), vestibular labyrinthitis/neuronitis, Mènière's disease, ototoxic drugs (e.g., gentamicin), acoustic schwannoma, trauma, compression of vestibular nerve

Central causes: Include CVA/TIA of brainstem, vertebral dissection, tumor, multiple sclerosis affecting brainstem/cerebellum

- Central causes may involve additional brainstem structures causing symptoms such as diplopia or dysphagia.

■ **Benign Positional Vertigo (BPV)**
- Otoliths moving in semicircular canals cause vertigo
- Can be preceded by viral illness
- No hearing loss

Treatment: Head movements recreate symptoms, lasting seconds to minutes

- Dix-Hallpike maneuver may be positive in BPV
- Meclizine may be tried but is often not effective
- Teach Epley maneuver in attempt to move otoliths and relieve symptoms

■ Mènière's Disease[10]
• Tinnitus, deafness, vertigo
• Typically, vertigo lasts hours and hearing worsens with vertigo

Pathophysiology: Rupture of the membranous labyrinth → endolymph mixes with perilymph

Treatment: Diuretics, eliminate ETOH/caffeine, salt restriction

• Labyrinthectomy (sacrifices hearing), vestibular neurectomy (preserves hearing)
• Direct injection of gentamycin into the middle ear

CENTRAL HEARING ABNORMALITIES

■ Auditory Agnosia
Right temporal lobe lesion

• Inability to interpret sounds

■ Amusia
Right temporal lobe lesion
• Inability to interpret music

BRAINSTEM AUDITORY EVOKED RESPONSES (BAERS) (SEE TABLE 4-1)
Average of a series of potentials generated from the major processing centers of the auditory system in response to a repetitive sound stimulus

• Sample lesion and effects include acoustic neuroma (retrocochlear) → prolonged I–III and I–V interpeak latencies; cochlear lesions → progressive disappearance at high-intensity stimulation of the interaural difference in the latency of wave V

Table 4-1 Brainstem Auditory Evoked Potentials (BAERs)

Wave	Lesion
I	cochlear nerve
II	cochlear nuclei (pons)
III	superior olivary complex (pons)
IV	lateral lemniscus (pons)
V	inferior colliculus (midbrain)
VI	medial geniculate (thalamus)
VII	auditory radiations

Table 4-2 Gardner Robertson Scale[11]

Grade	Description	Pure Tone Audiogram (dB)	Speech Discrimination (%)
I	good–excellent	0–30	70–100
II	serviceable	31–50	50–69
III	nonserviceable	51–90	5–49
IV	poor	91–max	1–4
V	none	not testable	0

NOTE: If pure tone audiogram and speech discrimination do not correlate, use the lower class

CHAPTER 5 ■ MOVEMENT DISORDERS[1-5]

Paul Kalanithi, MD

INTRODUCTION

Movement disorders are clinically characterized by involuntary movements, slowed movements, or inability to initiate movements. Major disease types are bradykinesias tremors, stereotypies, choreas, athetosis, and dystonias. The pathology of these diseases primarily involves the cortico-striato-thalamo-cortical circuits with principal focus on the basal ganglia (BG). The cortex is the major input, and the globus pallidus interna outputs to the thalamus. The classic circuit is depicted in Figure 5-1, though more recent models of BG function are considerably more complex and may employ oscillatory state, rather than firing rate.

TREMOR[6]

Tremors can be divided into resting tremors (more common) and action tremors (intention tremors and postural tremors). Resting tremors generally reflect basal ganglia pathology, while action tremors generally reflect cerebellar dysfunction. Severe action tremor can be caused by midbrain lesions, known as peduncular tremor. Some tremors can be treated with stereotactic surgery. Tremors generally increase with stress, fatigue, and certain exacerbating medications.

Types

- Parkinsonian: Pill rolling, resting, 3–6 Hz, extrapyramidal due to disease of basal ganglia and substantia nigra, remits during sleep
- Cerebellar: Intention tremor
- Benign essential tremor: familial, may involve the head ("yes-yes, no-no" movement)
- Due to medical condition: Pheochromocytoma, hyperthyroidism, hypoglycemia, anxiety, Wilson's disease
- Adverse drug effect: lithium, caffeine, methylphenidate
- Postural tremor: Alcohol withdrawal
- Dystonic
- Psychogenic
- Toxic (e.g., mercury poisoning)
- Infectious (e.g., syphilis)

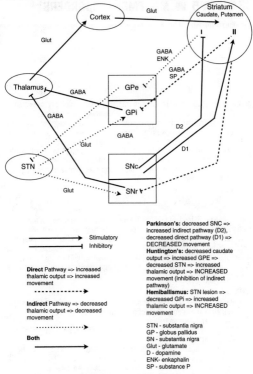

Figure 5-1 Diagrammatic representation of the connections between the cortex, striatum, and thalamus.

Treatment: Beta-blockers (propranolol), thalamotomy, thalamic stimulation, botulism toxin, Parkinson's medications, benzodiazepines (clonazepam), anti-seizure medications (primidone, gabapentin, topiramate), calcium channel blockers (nimodipine)

ESSENTIAL TREMOR

Clinical features: Tremor, usually of hands and forearms, worsened by movement, stress, anxiety

- Usual onset before age 30
- Improved with alcohol, propranolol

Pathophysiology: Unknown, may involve increased activity of inferior olives

Etiology: Usually familial

Medical treatment: Propranolol, primidone have best evidence. Other medications include topiramate, gabapentin and benzodiazepenes.

Surgical treatment: Thalamotomy or DBS of thalamus (Vim or dentatorubrothalamic tract) for severe cases; improves 90% of patients[7].

DYSTONIA

Localized slow contractions of specific muscle groups (local, segmental, or multifocal)

- Common localized dystonias include blepharospasm, torticollis, writer's cramp, and oral-facial dyskinesia
- Primary or secondary
- DDx includes drug reactions, encephalitis, stroke, toxicity, Lesch-Nyhan (X-linked), DYT1 (AD), dentatorubropallidoluysial atrophy (AD), Wilson's disease (AR), Hallervorden-Spatz disease (AR), mitochondrial disease
- Treatment may include botulinum injections, anticholinergics, benzodiazepines, anticonvulsants, lithium, reserpine, baclofen, levodopa

TORTICOLLIS AKA CERVICAL DYSTONIA[8]

Clinical features: Sustained, involuntary muscular contractions of cervical musculature, often causing abnormal postures of the head

Table 5-1 Tremor

Tremor	Frequency	Amplitude	Details
Parkinsonian	4–8 Hz	Variable	Worse at rest
Essential	4–8 Hz	Variable	Worse with action, stress
Physiologic	10–12 Hz	Low	Awake and asleep
Intention	2–3 Hz	Variable	Irregular

- Progresses from spasmodic to continual
- May be painful
- Generally affects adults (most prevalent in the 5th decade)

Etiology: May be genetic (loci on chromosomes 8 and 18), post-traumatic, or drug-induced (dopamine antagonists)

Pathophysiology: Unknown, may involve abnormal dopamine signaling, copper or manganese levels, neural plasticity

- Structures affected may be putamen, GPi (decreased thalamic inhibition by internal segment of globus pallidus leads to incomplete muscle relaxation), thalamus, midbrain, motor cortex, etc.
- Lesion of subthalamic nucleus may lead to dystonia or hemiballismus

Treatment: Periodic botulinum toxin injections, physical therapy, upper cervical ventral rhizotomies, spinal accessory neurectomy, stereotactic thalamotomy, microvascular decompression of spinal accessory nerve, myotomy

HEMIBALLISMUS

Symptoms: Violent, involuntary, flinging movement of extremity

Pathophysiology: Vascular infarct or destruction (e.g., hemorrhage) of the subthalamic nucleus or connections to globus pallidus

Treatment: Dopamine antagonists, antipsychotics, ventrolateral thalamotomy if refractory or persistent

Prognosis: Usually self limited and will resolve after 2 months

HYPOKINETIC DISORDERS

PARKINSON'S DISEASE[9-11]

Clinical features: Asymmetric symptoms at onset, bradykinesia, akinesia, "pill rolling" resting tremor (3–5 Hz), which remits during sleep, "cog-wheel" or "lead-pipe" rigidity, masked facies, postural instability, festinating gait, dementia (30%), depression

Epidemiology: 1% of population, peak incidence in 6th decade, M > F

Pathophysiology: Loss of dopaminergic neurons (80% to become symptomatic) in the substantia nigra (pars compacta) $\rightarrow$ overactivity of indirect basal ganglia circuit and underactivity of direct circuit of basal ganglia $\rightarrow$ causing decreased motor circuit activity (voluntary movement)

- Bradykinesia may be correlated with increased beta-band (10–30 Hz) activity in the Cd, Pt, and STN
- Resting tremor appears related to cerebellar inputs to thalamic nuclei

Etiology: Primarily idiopathic

- May involve mitochondrial dysfunction (decreased complex I activity), with increased alpha-synuclein and ubiquitin activity
- Toxic exposure may play a role

Medical treatment: Primarily dopamine agonism

- Levodopa (L-dopa) crosses into CNS where it is converted into dopamine; carbidopa (Sinemet) inhibits dopa decarboxylase to prevent systemic conversion into dopamine
- COMT (Catechol-O-Methyl Transferase) inhibitors (entacapone, tolapone) prevent metabolism of L-dopa
- Dopamine agonists (bromocriptine, pergolide)
- Monoamine oxidase B inhibitors (selegiline)
- Amantadine releases dopamine
- Anticholinergics (benzhexol, benztropin, artane)

Surgical treatment: See Functional Neurosurgery Chapter 16

- DBS of STN and GPi are used for patients with intolerable medication side effects, though some data indicates earlier surgery may be of significant benefit
- Best for tremor (Vim, unilateral only), dyskinesia, bradykinesia (STN)

CHAPTER 6 ■ INFECTIOUS DISEASES OF THE CENTRAL NERVOUS SYSTEM

Viet Nguyen, MD

BRAIN ABSCESS[1]

Local cerebritis with necrosis and surrounding edema encapsulated by fibroblasts and inflammatory cells

Etiology: Hematogenous spread (25%), local spread (50%), meningitis

Risk factors: Penetrating head trauma, open skull fracture, diabetes, alcohol abuse, immunosuppression, poor dentition, congenital heart disease, valvular infection, or implanted foreign body (ventricular drain, deep brain stimulator)

Symptoms/Signs: Headache (75%), fever (50%), altered mental status (50%)

DDx: Neoplasm (primary or metastatic), subacute stroke, radiation necrosis, resolving hematoma, HSV encephalitis, ADEM

Radiology: MRI (most sensitive) is bright on DWI, dark necrosis surrounded by bright edema on T2, ring-enhancing mass on T1 with gadolinium contrast

- CT shows hypodense necrotic core, but contrast ring-enhancement only after 2 wks (capsular formation)

Laboratory: Elevated peripheral WBC count, elevated ESR; blood cultures are less sensitive but still should be done

- AVOID lumbar puncture: Risk of herniation is higher than with other mass lesions; CSF cultures rarely elicit the organism
- Most common isolate is *Strep milleri*, many are polymicrobial

Complications: Mass effect, increased ICP, hydrocephalus, meningitis, papilledema, seizures, SIADH, diabetes insipidus, temperature dysregulation, local mass effect, and rarely, vasculitis and stroke

Outcomes: Mortality in adults 10–15%, children 25%

- Poor prognostic factors include stupor/coma (60–100% mortality), and rupture into a ventricle (80–100% mortality)

Treatment: IV antibiotics x 4–8 wks (as guided by follow-up imaging) and biopsy (to disrupt capsule and guide antibiotic therapy)

Table 6-1 IV Antibiotic Choice Is Based on Suspected Source

Suspected Source	Likely Organism	Treatment
empiric (unknown)		Ceftazidime (3rd-gen, 2g q8h) + Metronidazole (500 mg q6h)
middle ear mastoid	strep, pseudomonas, bacteriodes, enterobacter	Metronidazole (15 mg/kg load, followed by 7.5 mg/kg q6–8h) + Cefepime (4th-gen, 2g q6h) OR Meropenem (2g q8h)
nasopharynx sinuses teeth	strep, bacteriodes, proteus, staph aureus, hemophilus, anaerobes, Mucor	Metronidazole (15 mg/kg load, followed by 7.5 mg/kg q6–8h) + Penicillin-G (4 million units q4h) OR Ceftriaxone (3rd-gen, 2 g q12h) OR Cefotaxime (3rd-gen, 2 g q4–6h)
penetrating head trauma	staph aureus, strep, enterobacter, clostridium	Nafcillin OR Oxacillin (2g q4h) OR Vancomycin (15 mg/kg q12h) PLUS Ceftriaxone (3rd-gen, 2 g q12h) OR Cefotaxime (3rd-gen, 2 g q4–6h)
postoperative neurosurgical		Vancomycin (15 mg/kg q12h) PLUS Cefepime (3rd-gen, 2 g q8h)
AIDS	Toxoplama*, fungi	Pyrimethamine (PO 200 mg load, followed by 75–100 mg/day) + Sulfadiazine (PO 1–1.5 g 4x/day, given with pyrimethamine and folinic acid) OR Clindamycin (PO 450 mg 4x/day or 600 mg PO/IV q6h) MRSA: Linezolid 600 mg q12h

*Tunkel[4]

- Surgical removal only if loculated, enlarging despite proper antibiotic therapy, or impending herniation
- Steroids only if needed for reducing edema or ICP (Dexamethasone IV 10 mg load, followed by 4 mg q6h)

SUBDURAL EMPYEMA[2]

Rapid spread of pus over the brain surface

Etiology: Local infectious spread

Risk factors: Frontal/ethmoid sinusitis, skull fracture, venous sinus thrombosis, penetrating head trauma, craniotomy

Symptoms/Signs: Headache, localized pain, fever, partial (and secondary generalized) seizures, AMS

DDx: Subdural hematoma, meningioma, granuloma (TB/sarcoid)

Radiology: CT with contrast shows hypodense crescent-shaped collection molding the cortex with enhancing margins

- MRI shows T1-hyperintense and T2-isointense-to-CSF collection which can cross fossae boundaries (unlike epidural abscess)
- Infection/enhancement tracks along the interhemispheric fissure/ convexities

CSF: Lumbar puncture not recommended, but if done, shows mild lymphocytic pleocytosis, increased protein, normal glucose

Treatment: Surgical drainage (send gram stain and culture for organisms), debridement of extracranial source, antibiotics x 4–6 wks (choice based on organism and course determined by clinical and radiographic response)

Outcome: Prognosis excellent when recognized and treatment rendered early

SPINE INFECTION

OSTEOMYELITIS[3]

Etiology: Infection of bone, usually by pyogenic bacteria and mycobacteria

- Pus buildup raises intraosseous pressure, impairing blood flow
- Chronic ischemia and necrosis form a sequestrum; periosteum deposits new bone around it
- Often not diagnosed until chronic. History and exam confounded by the original trauma, overlying soft tissue infection, or baseline degenerative bone disease
- Hematogenous spread, local soft tissue spread, or directly from trauma or surgery

Risk factors: Trauma, IV drug use, ischemia, foreign bodies, concurrent infection in another site with or without bacteremia

Location: Vertebral bodies (highly vascular) affected in adults

- Affects lumbar (50%) > thoracic (35%) > cervical (15%) spine, except in tuberculous spondylitis (Pott's disease), where the thoracic spine is most commonly affected
- Long bones affected in children, where the metaphysis of growing bones is well perfused

Symptoms/Signs: Acute or subacute illness with fever, chills, dull localized pain and tenderness, decreased painful range of movement (spasm of the paraspinal muscles), or painful weight-bearing

- Local erythema and soft tissue swelling
- Nerve root irritation can cause atypical pain in the chest, abdomen, or extremity

Complications: Epidural abscess

- Failure to recognize epidural abscess before neurologic deficits develop can cause irreversible paralysis

Radiology: MRI is the best diagnostic procedure; should be performed in all cases of vertebral osteomyelitis accompanied by subjective weakness or objective spinal cord abnormalities to rule out epidural abscess

- Plain radiographs → soft-tissue swelling (early), periosteal reaction (> 10-day lag from onset of infection), lytic changes (after 2–6 weeks)
- CT or MRI: Epidural, paraspinal, retropharyngeal, mediastinal, retroperitoneal, or psoas abscesses that originate in the spine
- 99Tc-monodiphosphonate bone scan: High sensitivity but low specificity, especially with underlying bone abnormalities
- MRI: High sensitivity and specificity; fat-suppressed T1-weighted postgadolinium images show affected vertebral bodies although gadolinium may not be necessary if are uses STIR, as well as any involved disks and inflammatory soft tissue; can alert to compression of the thecal sac; need to distinguish from healing fractures and tumors

Laboratory: Increased erythrocyte sedimentation rate (ESR) and C-reactive protein (CRP) level

- Can also have normal or modestly elevated white blood cell count, anemia
- Blood cultures indicated in acute cases, less sensitive in chronic disease (20–50%)

Treatment: Antibiotics (see Table 6–2)

Table 6-2 Antibiotic Selection for the Treatment of Osteomyelitis

Gram Stain	Organism	Antibiotic
Gram-positive	MSSA	*Nafcillin* or *Cefazolin* or *Ceftriaxone* or *Clindamycin*
Gram-positive	MRSA	*Vancomycin* + *Rifampin*; or *Clindamycin* or *Linezolid* or *Daptomycin*
Gram-positive	Streptococci	*Penicillin* or *Cefazolin* or *Ceftriaxone* or *Clindamycin*
Gram-negative	Escherichia coli	*Ampicillin* or *Cefazolin* or *Ceftriaxone Ciprofloxacin IV/PO*
Gram-negative	Pseudomonas aeruginosa	*(Piperacillin/Tazobactam; or Ceftazidime) + Tobramycin*
Gram-negative	Enterobacter	*Piperacillin/Tazobactam* or *Ceftazidime* or *Ciprofloxacin*
	Anaerobes/mixed	*Ampicillin/Sulbactam* or *Piperacillin/Tazobactam* or a carbapenem; or *Ciprofloxacin* + *Clindamycin* or *Metronidazole*

Osteomyelitis Antibiotic Doses:

Antibiotic	Dose
Ampicillin	2 g IV q4h
Ampicillin/Sulbactam	1.5–3g IV q6h
Cefazolin	1g IV q8h
Ceftazidime	2g IV q12h
Ceftriaxone	1g IV q24h
Ciprofloxacin	400 mg IV, or 750 mg PO q12h
Clindamycin	900 mg IV q8h
Daptomycin	4–6mg/kg IV q24h
Linezolid	600 mg IV/PO q12h
Metronidazole	500 mg PO tid
Nafcillin	2g IV q4h
Penicillin	3–4 million U IV q4h
Piperacillin/Tazobactam	3.375 g IV q6h
Rifampin	300 mg PO q12h
Tobramycin	5–7 mg/kg q24h
Vancomycin	15 mg/kg IV q12h

- Fluoroscopy, ultrasound, or CT-guided needle aspiration of pus or bone biopsy for culture and sensitivities to guide antibiotic therapy (if culture not simply done at debridement)
- Surgery in cases of spinal instability, new or progressive neurologic deficits, or large soft-tissue abscesses that cannot be drained otherwise; debridement to remove necrotic bone and abnormal soft tissues; epidural abscesses should be surgically drained
- Optimize nutritional and metabolic status to promote healing
- Anecdotal-level data for: Prolonged oral antibiotic therapy (esp. with foreign body), hyperbaric oxygen, antibiotic-impregnated methacrylate beads in chronic osteomyelitis

Duration of Therapy

Children: 4–6 weeks (< 3 weeks = 10 x greater failure rate)

Adults 6–8 weeks; consider longer if ESR does not decrease by 2/3s or CRP does not normalize

SPINAL EPIDURAL ABSCESS[5]

Etiology: Hematogenous spread

Symptoms: Spine tenderness, fever, pain

Risk factors: Immunocompromised, IV drugs, diabetes, postoperative, hemodialysis, alcoholism

Radiology: On MRI, hyperintense on T2 with contrast enhancement

Laboratory: Cultures frequently show staph aureus

Treatment: Surgery for decompression, debridement and for diagnostic cultures
- IV antibiotics for 6–8 weeks

OTHER

DISCITIS (PYOGENIC SPONDYLITIS)

Common organisms: Staph aureus >>> Enterobacter, E. coli, Pseudomonas, klebsiella
- Seed hematogenously, or directly from adjacent areas

Symptoms: Fever, pain

Labs: Elevated ESR, CRP, may have positive blood cultures

POTT'S DISEASE (TUBERCULOSIS IN THE SPINE)

- If spine is unstable, the management is surgery followed by 6 months of IV antibiotics
- If spine is stable, then get an IR-guided biopsy to confirm TB and then administer 6 months of IV antibiotics (Rifampin, Isoniazide/B_{12}, etc.)
- ID consult is mandatory
- Follow CRP/SED rates

II. NEUROSURGERY

Griffith Harsh, MD
Michael SB Edwards, MD

CHAPTER 7 ■ PEDIATRIC NEUROSURGERY[1]

Kevin Chao, MD

Melanie G. Hayden Gephart, MD, MAS

Early embryo development:
morula ⇒ blastocyst ⇒ embryoblast (⇒ epiblast ⇒ yolk sac, embryo),
trophoblast (cytotrophoblast, syncytiotrophoblast ⇒ placenta)

NEUROLOGICAL EXAMINATION OF INFANTS AND TODDLERS[2]

NEWBORN

General: Spontaneous, smooth movements, attentive, responsive to light

Cranial nerves: Crying (VII, IX, X), suck and swallow (V, VII, IX, X, XII), eye movement (II, III, IV, VI), light response (II, III), sound response (VIII)

Tone: Resting flexed posture, arm traction (grasp wrist/ankle and pull until shoulder/hip is off the mat → continued flexion at the elbow/knee), arm/leg recoil (arms/legs extended then quickly released → should return to flexion), hand position as a fist, head lag

Positions: Prone (should be able to turn head side to side), ventral suspension (head should be the same level as back), vertical suspension (holding hands under arms, baby should not slip through)

Reflexes: Hyperreflexia can be normal, ankle and patellar are easiest to elicit, plantar (toes upgoing), suck, root, Moro, stepping, grasp

3 MONTHS

General: Attentive, tracks, social smile, frowns

Cranial nerves: Vestibulo-ocular reflex, full facial expression

Motor: Decreased flexor tone, more open hand, will hold object but cannot reach, regards hand, slight head lag

Positions: Supine (spontaneous movement), prone (can bring head up 45–90°, weight borne on forearms), vertical suspension (can support some weight with legs)

NORMAL INFANT REFLEXES[3]

Table 7-1 Normal Neonatal/Infant Reflexes Appearance/Disppearance

Reflex (description)	Appears	Disappears
Moro - lift head 30° and let fall to neutral. A positive test = arm extension and abduction, then arm adduction	Birth	1-3 months
Palmar grasp - object in hand causes flexion/ grasping	Birth	4 months
Root response - stroking cheek causes mouth to turn in direction of stimulus	Birth	3-4 months
Tonic neck - turn head to side while child is supine, with ipsilateral arm & leg extending and opposite arm/leg flexing. Normal infant tries to break reflex position	Birth	5-6 months
+ Babinski - stroking lateral border of sole, to big toe. A positive reflex causes big toe dorsiflexion, and fanning of other toes	Birth	1-2 years

Reflexes: Crossed adductor can be normal (should not persist beyond 7 months), root (disappears at 4 months), moro (disappears at 4–5 months), grasp (disappears at 4–6 months for hands, 12 months for toes)

6 MONTHS

General: Social awareness, laughs, smiles, jabbers, repetitive and nonspecfic sounds

Cranial nerves: Visually tracks, hearing, facial movement

Motor: Sits, reaches for objects, brings to midline and into mouth, works well with both hands, raking grasp, actively pulls to sitting position, rolls over front to back

Position: Prone (brings chest off the mat), vertical suspension (baby fully supports weight)

Reflexes: Landau (postural reflex; head in flexion → legs in flexion, head released, legs and head return to extension), propping, parachute (arms extend to catch self)

12 MONTHS

General: Stranger anxiety, imitates, waves bye-bye, follows simple instructions, feeds self, speaks one or two words

Cranial nerves: Ocular range of motion, visual fields

Reflexes: Parachute

Table 7-2 Neuroembryology Stage and Clinical Correlate

Postovulatory Week	Stage	Neurodevelopment	Clinical Correlate
0–8	**Embryonic**		
1	Implantation	Blastocyst	Miscarriage
2	Germ layer separation	Formation of neural plate	Enterogenous cyst fistula, split notochord syndrome
3–4	Dorsal induction (aka primary neurulation)	Folding of the neural plate leading to the neural groove and tube/crest, closure of neuropores, paired alar plates, neural tube forms and closes, three primary neuromeres of brain form**	Spinal + cranial dysraphism*, chiari II malformation
4	Secondary neurulation	Formation of the caudal neural tube from the caudal eminence	Sacral agenesis, caudal regression syndromes
4–6	Ventral induction (aka telencephalization)	Formation of the cerebral hemispheres, eyes, olfactory bulb/tract, pituitary gland, part of face	Holoprosencephaly, Dandy-Walker malformation, craniosynostosis
9–24	**Fetal**	**Formation of cortical plate**	
6–16	Neurogenesis	Neuronal/glial proliferation and apoptosis	Micro- and megalencephaly
12–24	Migration	Cortical neuron migration and formation of corpus callosum	Agenesis of corpus callosum, failure of frontal lobe development, neuronal migration disorders***
24–40	**Perinatal**	**Neuronal maturation**	
24–birth	Organization	Migration, organization, maturation synaptogenesis	Cortical dysplasias
Birth–2 years	Myelination	Myelination	Disorders of myelination

* includes anencephaly, encephalocele, myelomeningocele, myeloschisis
** includes prosencephalon, mesencephalon, rhombencephalon
*** includes lissencephaly, polymicrogyria, schizencephaly, heterotopia

Table 7-3 Embryologic Milestones

Gestational Age (days)	Embryologic Event
4	12–16 blastomeres, morula forming
7–14	Embryonic implantation; formation of three germ layers; bilaminar disc → epiblast and hypoblast
13	Formation of primitive streak
17	Formation of notochord
22	Fusion of folds to form neural tube; neural crest development
24	Closure of cranial neuropore (lamina terminalis)
26	Closure of caudal neuropore
4th week	Dilations and folding of rostral neural tube; formation of prosencephalon, mesencephalon, and rhombencephalon
5th week	Prosencephalon → telencephalon and diencephalon → cerebrum and basal ganglia Mesencephalon → (does not divide) → midbrain Rhombencephalon → metencephalon and myelencephalon → pons and medulla

Motor: Pincer grasp, follows commands, transitions in and out of sitting, creeping, crawling, cruising, walk (11–14 months)

18 MONTHS

General: Expresses wants, vocabulary of 10+ words, follows commands, understands function of objects, points

Cranial nerves: Conjugate eye movement, near reflex, facial movement

Motor: Objects in cup, stacks blocks, pincer grasp, draws, overhand throw of ball, walks

2.5 YEARS

General: Socially interactive, plays, follows commands, names objects, responds to questions, four-word sentences with pronouns and plurals, names body parts, stacks blocks, draws

Motor: Throws and kicks ball, walks, runs

NEURAL TUBE DEVELOPMENT

Prior to implantation, the inner cell mass of the blastocyst converts into an epiblast and hypoblast (will form the endoderm). From the epiblast, the mesoderm appears near day 21. Formation of the primitive streak (linear thickening on the dorsal surface of the epiblast) at the caudal end signifies the beginning of gastrulation. Hensen's node is at the cephalic end of the primitive streak and contains the primitive pit. Cells migrate into the primitive pit and form the notochord (from mesoderm). Ectoderm overlies the notochord and consists of germinal matrix, mangle, and marginal zones. The ectoderm differentiates into neural ectoderm, forming the neural plate. The neural plate elongates in a rostro-caudal direction. Neural folds arise laterally and fuse to form the neural tube. The fusion starts at the caudal rhombencephalon and progresses rostral and caudal (aka primary neurulation). Errors in primary neurulation lead to spinal dysraphism (e.g., spina bifida, anencephaly).

Table 7-4 Major Neuroembryologic and Mature Structures

Embryologic Structure	Adult Derivative
Neural tube/plate (from ectoderm)	Cortical neurons, spinal cord, brain, all preganglionic autonomic fibers, all fibers innervating skeletal muscles
Neural crest (lateral folds of the neural plate)	Adrenal medulla, dorsal root ganglia of cranial and spinal nerves, pigmented layers of retina, sympathetic ganglia of autonomic nervous system, peripheral nervous system, viscero- and neurocranium, pia, arachnoid, endocrine cells
Mesoderm	Dura, connective tissue investments of peripheral nerve fibers (endoneurium, perineurium, epineurium)
Diencephalon	Globus pallidus, 3rd ventricle, optic chiasm, optic nerves, infundibulum, mammillary eminences
Telencephalon	Amygdala, caudate, claustrum, putamen, cerebral hemispheres, olfactory bulbs, lateral ventricles
Rhombencephalon (primary vesicle) → metencephalon, myelencephalon (secondary vesicle)	Hindbrain, cerebellum, pons, medulla, 4th ventricle
Prosencephalon	Forebrain, optic vesicles, telencephalic (lateral) and diencephalic (3rd) ventricles
Mesencephalon	Midbrain, cerebral aqueduct
Caudal cell mass of neural tube	Sacral spinal cord, vertebra caudal to S2
Alar plate* (of neural tube)	Sensory neurons (GSA, GVA) in brainstem and spinal cord, dorsal horn
Basal plate (of neural tube)	Motor neurons (GSE, GVE), ventral horn
Somites	Vertebral column, dorsal spine musculature
Notochord	Intervertebral discs
Floor plate	Ventral white commissure
Otic placode	Organ of corti/spiral ganglion, cristae ampullares, maculae utriculi/sacculi, vestibular ganglion, vestibulocochlear nerve

* Sulcus limitans divides the alar and basal plate

DEVELOPMENTAL DELAY

DDx of developmental delay: Down syndrome, autistic spectrum disorder, Fragile X syndrome, Prader-Willi/Angelman syndrome, Rett syndrome, inborn error of metabolism, Landau-Kleffner syndrome, neuronal migration disorders, social/environmental factors (abuse/neglect, malnutrition)

- Frequently multifactorial

Diagnostic evaluation: Careful pre-/perinatal, developmental, and social history

- Review of newborn screening results
- Hearing/vision screen
- Imaging: MRI brain in select cases
- Labs: Lead level, T4/TSH, high-resolution chromosomes, serum amino acids, urine organic acids

MACROCEPHALY AND MICROCEPHALY[4]

Head circumference (HC): Full-term (38–40 week) infant → 35 cm
- 3 mos → 40 cm
- 9 mos → 45 cm
- 3 yrs → 50 cm
- 9 yrs → 55 cm
- 3-9-5 rule helpful (increase circumference 5 cm between birth, 3 and 9 months, 3 and 9 years)

MACROCEPHALY

> 2 standard deviations above mean HC
- Due to one of three mechanisms: Too much fluid (hydrocephalus), too much brain (megalencephaly), too much blood (hematoma)

DDx: Hydrocephalus (communicating and noncommunicating), Chiari malformations (secondary to hydrocephalus), arachnoid cyst, benign extra-axial fluid of infancy, subdural hematoma or hygroma, familial (benign) macrocephaly (large parental head size), Fragile X syndrome, neurocutaneous syndromes (e.g., NF, TS), holoprosencephaly, Alexander disease, Canavan disease, achondroplasia

Diagnostic evaluation: Thorough history and exam should narrow diagnosis, measure parents' head size, neuroimaging (ultrasound, CT, then MRI)

MICROCEPHALY

< 2 standard deviations below mean HC
- Usually secondary to underlying disorder
- Always consider in context of gestational age, body weight, and height

DDx: Intrauterine injury/ischemic stroke (illicit drugs, malnutrition, TORCH infection)

- Chromosomal anomalies (Trisomy 21, 13, 18)
- Inborn errors of metabolism (PKU, maple-syrup urine disease)
- Maternal diabetes mellitus
- Craniosynostosis
- Syndromes of dysmorphogenesis (Prader-Willi, Angelman, Rett)
- Protein storage and folding (Batten disease, Pelizaeus-Merzbacher disease)
- Neuronal migration disorders (lissencephaly, polymicrogyria, holoprosencephaly)

Diagnostic evaluation: Thorough history and exam including height and weight should narrow diagnosis

- High-resolution chromosomes
- Neuroimaging: MRI preferred over CT except in case of suspected craniosynostosis or TORCH infection
- Labs: Serum amino acids, urine organic acids; newborns should also undergo tox screen of serum, urine, and stool
- Infectious workup, including CSF studies, as indicated for suspected TORCH infections

■ **TORCH Infections**

Infectious entities with maternal to fetal transmission
- Classically includes toxoplasma (hydrocephalus, bilateral chorioretinitis, cranial calcifications), rubella (cortical/basal ganglia calcifications), cytomegalovirus (periventricular calcifications, microcephaly), herpes simplex 1 and 2, HIV
- Mother frequently asymptomatic

INTRACRANIAL HEMORRHAGE[2]

GERMINAL MATRIX HEMORRHAGE

Main cause of intracranial hemorrhage in *premature* neonates (< 34 weeks, low birth weight)

- Risk factors include perinatal distress, asphyxia, immaturity
- Can occur prenatally (See Table 7-5)

Table 7-5 Grading of Subependymal Germinal Matrix Hemorrhage

I	confined to germinal matrix
II	extension into adjacent lateral ventricle
III	interventricular hemorrhage with hydrocephalus
IV	hemorrhage in periventricular white matter with hydrocephalus, infarct, compression of deep medullary veins (90% mortality)

Table 7-6 CSF Shunt Obstruction - Predictive Score

Early Presenters (within 5 months of surgery)		Late Presenters (> 9 months to 2 years since surgery)	
Clinical Feature	Points	Clinical Feature	Points
Fluid tracking around shunt	1	Nausea & vomiting	1
Headache	1	Loss of developmental milestones	1
Irritability	1		
Fever	1	↑ Head circumference	1
Bulging fontanelle	2	Fluid tracking around shunt	1
Erythema at surgery site	3	↓ Level of consciousness	3
↓ Level of consciousness	3		

Early shunt score (total points above)	Shunt Failure Probability	Late shunt score (total points above)	Shunt Failure Probability
0 points	4%	0 points	8%
1 point	50%	1 point	38%
2 points	75%	≥ 2 points	100%
≥ 3 points	100%		

Other features (not found to be independent predictors of shunt failure) include inability to depress or refill CSF reservoir, papilledema, cranial nerve palsy, abd. pain/mass, meningismus and peritonitis
J Neurosurg 2001;94:202

Table 7-7 CSF Shunt Infections - Presenting Features in Children

Feature	V-P Shunt[*]	V-A Shunt[*]	Most Common Organisms	
Fever	95%	100%	Staph epidermidis (SE)	32–57%
Shunt malfunction	57%	14%	Staph. aureus (SA)	4–38%
Abdominal pain	48%	0	SA + Strep. viridans	4–15%
Meningismus	29%	0	Gram negatives ± SE	15% (3%)
Headache	14%	14%	SE + Enterococcus	7%
Irritability	19%	43%	SE + Strep. pyogenes	4%
Nephritis	0	14%	Enterococcus/Candida	4%

* V-A – ventriculoatrial, V-P – ventriculoperitoneal
Infection 1993;21:89; *Pediatr Neurosurg* 1999;30:253

Pathophysiology: Hypoxic injury to microcirculation of germinal matrix → loss of autoregulation → overperfusion → hemorrhage

Symptoms: Respiratory distress (hyaline membrane disease), coagulopathy, congenital heart disease, hypernatremia

CHOROID PLEXUS HEMORRHAGE

Most common cause of interventricular hemorrhage in *term* neonate
- Symptoms range from asymptomatic to hydrocephalus and increased intracranial pressure

TENTORIAL OR POSTERIOR FOSSA HEMORRHAGE

Etiology: Tearing of bridging veins along the posterior falx and tentorium
- Occurs in full-term, large birth weight baby, precipitous delivery

HYPOXIC-ISCHEMIC FETAL LESIONS

PORENCEPHALY

Pathology: Smooth-walled cyst wedges extending from the ventricle lined by gliotic white matter

Etiology: Ischemic insult to normally developed fetal brain

Radiology: Generally adjacent to sylvian fissure/central sulci, symmetric

Symptoms/Signs: Mental retardation, congenital hemiplegia, chronic spasticity, epilepsy

VENTRICULOPERITONEAL SHUNT (VPS)

INDICATIONS

Diversion of CSF flow, generally from hydrocephalus (communicating or obstructive) but also can be for other intracranial pathology. Alternatives to a peritoneal shunt include pleural or atrial.Shunt malfunction rate generally 5% (malfunction and infection most common) but up to 17%

VPS MALFUNCTION
SHUNT MALFUNCTION WORKUP AND MANAGEMENT

History: Reason for shunt insertion, last revision date and reason, last access of shunt, any recent abdominal infections/symptoms presence of accessory hardware, type and setting (pressure) of shunt, symptoms with last shunt malfunction/infection, sick contacts, baseline neurological status

Symptoms: Headache, nausea, vomiting, diplopia, lethargy, ataxia, irritability, seizures, swelling around shunt

Physical Exam: Increased head circumference (track OFC plot), full fontanelle, splayed sutures, papilledema, CSF around shunt tract, pseudomeningocele, ability of shunt reservoir to pump and refill (difficult to depress → distal obstruction)

- Slow to refill → proximal obstruction; not universal and only a small volume moves with each tap, so if refilling easily, do not be falsely reassured that the shunt is working properly). If shunt malfunction is severe, can lead to bradycardia, hemodynamic instability, and death (refractory ventricular arrhythmias). Be sure to include ear, throat, abdominal exam

Workup: Noncontrast HCT (compare to priors; remember, children with shunt malfunction/infection may not always have increased ventricular size), shunt tap if infection suspect or to evaluate proximal control/temporize (send for CSF gram stain/culture/protein/glucose/cell count with differential), shunt series (XR including AP skull, lateral skull, AP neck, chest, abd)

INDICATIONS FOR SHUNT TAP

1. Obtain CSF specimen (e.g., evaluate for infection)
2. Evaluate shunt function (proximal and distal flow, check pressure with manometer)
3. To inject medication (e.g., antibiotics or chemotherapy, but generally done via an ommaya reservoir)
4. Temporizing measure (remove CSF, prior to planned revision, to relieve increased intracranial pressure)

Treatment: Plan for urgent/emergent shunt revision, telemetry, If patient is moribund, may tap shunt to draw off CSF, or in extreme situations, access ventricle through shunt burr hole

■ Overshunting

Complications include slit ventricle syndrome (seen on head CT chronically in 12% of shunted children), intracranial hypotension, subdural hematomas, secondary craniosynostosis, aqueductal stenosis

Symptoms: Usually intermittent

- Nausea, vomiting, headache, lethargy, diplopia, upward gaze palsy, improves when patient prostrates
- Slow filling of shunt valve

Treatment: Watchful waiting (many spontaneously get better), shunt revision (choose valve with higher resistance) or increasing shunt setting (if an adjustable valve), 3rd ventriculostomy

PEDIATRIC SPINE

Table 7-8 Maturation of the Spine

Vertebrae	Primary Ossification Centers	Age at Presentation	Age at Closure Neurocentral Synchondrosis (Laminae)
C1	1 Anterior arch 2 Neural arches	20% at birth 80% 6–12 mon Birth	5–7 yr (3–4 yr)
C2	1 Body 2 Neural arches 1 Odontoid	Birth Birth Birth	3–6 yr (3–6 yr)
C3–L5	1 Body 2 Neural arches	Birth	3–6 yr (1–3 yr)
	Secondary Ossification Centers		**Ossification Completed**
C2	Odontoid apex (os terminale)	2–6 yr	Fuses with body of dens by 12 yr
C3–L5	Superior articulating facets Inferior articulating facets Transverse processes Spinous processes	10–13 yr	18–25 yr
C3–L5	Ring apophyses	10–13 yr	18–25 yr

NOTE: Overall adult spine configuration around age 8–12 years

SPINAL DYSRAPHISM (NEURAL TUBE DEFECTS [NTD])

Includes spina bifida occulta spectrum, meningocele, myelomeningocele, myelocystocele, myeloschisis

▉ Spina Bifida Aperta
(Cystica, "open" NTD)
  Includes meningocele, myelomeningocele, myeloschisis (rachischisis)

Epidemiology: 0.1–0.2% incidence, F > M

Etiology: Lack of neural fold fusion → neural placode
  • Failed dysjunction → midline cutaneous defects

Location: Lumbosacral > thoracolumbar > isolated lumbar

▉ Meningocele
Cystic dilation of meninges herniating through posterior or anterior bony defects
  • Neural elements (e.g., spinal cord) normal
  • Associated with hydrocephalus

■ Myelomeningocele

Midline vertebral bone defect through which meninges or neural placode is visible

- Associated with hydrocephalus, chiari II, syringomyelia, diastematomyelia, lipomas, dermoid and epidermoid cysts, ventral abnormalities, vertebral abnormalities

■ Myeloschisis (Rachischisis)

Flat mass of nervous tissue without overlying skin or membrane
- Most severe of spina bifida spectrum
- Not compatible with survival

■ Lipomyelomeningoceles

Extradural lipoma attached to neural placode with protrusion through posterior vertebral defects

- Associated with syringohydromyelia, tethered cord, cutaneous stigmata, vertebral anomalies, dural defects, sacral anomalies

Subtypes: Transitional, dorsal, terminal

Epidemiology: Most common occult spinal dysraphism

- F > M

Etiology: Error in separation of neuroectoderm from cutaneous ectoderm (disjunction) leading to mesoderm ventrally before the neural ectoderm has completely fused

Symptoms/Signs: Clinically obvious lumbosacral mass or sinus

- Usually asymptomatic
- May be detected following onset of symptoms of sensory loss, lower extremity weakness, neurogenic bladder

Location: Lumbosacral spine

Treatment: Surgical untethering of the spinal cord, resection of lipoma

■ Dermal Sinus Tract

Associated with hypertrichosis, capillary hemangioma, dermoid or epidermoid cysts, spinal lipoma

Etiology: Failure of focal disjunction

Pathology: Epithelial-lined connection of skin to spinal cord or filum terminale

Location: Cephalic or caudal end (lumbosacral) of neural tube, most commonly near S2

DDx: Pilonidal sinus tract (closer to anus, fibrous tract to coccyx)

Treatment: As risk for meningitis is high, tract must be resected

- Rule out intracranial or intraspinal mass (dermoid)

▨ Split-Cord Malformations[5–7]
Previously known as diastematomyelia
- Diplomyelia is true duplication of the spinal cord with two sets of motor and sensory roots

Error in secondary neurulation
- F > M
- Usually between T9 and S1
- Associated with cutaneous stigmata, hemi- or butterfly vertebra, intersegmental laminar fusion, intervertebral disc narrowing, scoliosis, narrowed disc space, syringomyelia
- 5% of scoliosis, 30% of myelomeningoceles

Type I Two hemicords, each in a separate dural tube, with the tube separated by a median bony septum

Treatment: Surgical untethering of the spinal cord, removing the bony septum, reconstructing a single dural tube

Type II Two hemicords within a single dural tube, separated by nonrigid fibrous septum

Treatment: Surgical untethering of the spinal cord

▨ Tethered Cord
Symptoms: Neurogenic bladder and bowel, incontinence, delay in toilet training, scoliosis, foot deformities, distal motor/sensory loss, unilateral limb atrophy

Pathology: Low lying conus, thickened filum terminale (1.5 mm), lateral/superior coursing nerve roots

DDx of Skin-Covered Lumbosacral Mass
Spinal lipoma, teratoma, simple meningocele

▨ Caudal Regression Syndrome[5,7]
Ranges from absent coccyx to complete lumbosacral agenesis
- Associated with renal dysplasia, imperforate anus, genitourinary malformation, dermoid tumors, myelomeningocele, clubfoot, cardiovascular anomalies, kyphosis, spina bifida occulta complex

Epidemiology: M = F
- Associated with maternal hyperglycemia

Caudal Agenesis Syndrome
Absent lower vertebrae, anal atresia, malformed genitalia, renal abnormalities, lower extremity maldevelopment, fusion of lower extremities (aka sirenomyelia)
- Associated with diabetic mothers (16%), diastematomyelia, intraspinal lipomas, dermoids, dermal sinuses, tethered cord

Symptoms/Signs: Neurogenic bladder, motor weakness, lower extremity deformities (caudal regression syndrome)

NEURENTERIC (ENTEROGENOUS) CYSTS[5,7]

Abnormal persistence of the neurenteric canal leads to an intradural extramedullary lesion lined with intestinal mucosa that can hemorrhage and result in spinal cord compression

- Associated with extraspinal cysts

Epidemiology: Present before young adulthood

Etiology: Failure of separation between notochord and foregut

Symptoms/Signs: Depends on location of lesion, but can include vertebral body abnormalities, ataxia, cranial nerve palsies, myelopathy, meningitis, pain

Pathology: Nucin-producing goblet cells

Location: Intraspinal >> intracranial

- Cervicothoracic or conus

CRANIOSYNOSTOSIS[5,8]

The premature closure of cranial sutures. Cranial sutures remain open until adulthood, except the metopic which closes by 2 years

Epidemiology: M > F (except unilateral coronal)

DDx: Positional flattening (positional plagiocephaly, brachycephaly)

Genetics: Fibroblast growth factor receptor mutation

- Turribrachycephaly → chromosome 7p

Workup: 3D reconstructed fine cut CT to evaluate suture closure

■ Kleeblattschadel
Fusion of multiple sutures → cloverleaf-shaped skull

Table 7-9 Craniosynostosis

Suture Closed	Percentage of Overall Synostoses	Head Shape
Sagittal	56–58%	Scaphocephaly
Bilateral Coronal	20–30%	Brachycephaly, oxycephaly, turricephaly; "harlequin eyes"
Metopic	5–20%	Trigonocephaly
Unilateral Coronal	10–20%	Plagiocephaly
Lambdoid	1–3%	Posterior plagiocephaly/pachycephaly

- Chromosome 15 q mutation of fibroblast growth factor receptor gene

Apert's Syndrome[9]

Craniosynostoses: Both coronal sutures (+/- other sutures)

Epidemiology: 5% of craniosynostosis

- 1/65,000 in general population

Symptoms/Signs: Hydrocephalus and mental retardation despite treatment (not universal), syndactyly, cleft palate, frontal encephalocele, prognathism, turribrachycephaly, multisystem anomalies (choanal stenoses/atresia), midfacial hypoplasia

Genetics: Autosomal dominant(AD)

- Keratinocyte growth factor receptor (KGFR)—mediated effect from missense substitution mutation

Outcome: Intelligence varies, but a significant percentage are mentally retarded despite treatment of hydrocephalus

Crouzon Syndrome

Craniosynostoses: Bilateral coronal, frontosphenoid, frontoethmoid

Symptoms/Signs: Hypertelorism, hydrocephalus, proptosis, midfacial hypoplasia ("parrot's beak"), maxillary hypoplasia, ear malformation, agenesis of corpus callosum

Genetics: Autosomal dominant

- Fibroblast GFR2 mutation

Outcome: Normal intelligence, fewer CNS anomalies than Pfeiffer or Apert

Pfeiffer Syndrome

Craniosynostoses: Coronal and lambdoid > sagittal

Subtypes: (1) Better prognosis; (2) cloverleaf skull; (3) turribrachycephaly

Symptoms/Signs: Midface hypoplasia, exophthalmos, ocular proptosis, hypertelorism, broad thumbs/toes, hydrocephalus, strabismus, hearing loss, choanal atresia/stenosis, laryngotracheal abnormalities, ankylosis skeletal abnormalities

Genetics: AD, complete penetrance, FGFR1,2 mutation

Saethre-Chotzen Syndrome

Craniosynostoses: Unilateral coronal

Genetics: TWIST mutation, AD, complete penetrance, variable expressivity

Symptoms/Signs: Low-set hairline, long ear crura, facial asymmetry, midfacial hypoplasia, limb abnormalities, developmental delay, hearing loss

■ Carpenter's Syndrome
Craniosynostoses: Sagittal, lambdoid

Genetics: Autosomal recessive (AR), unknown gene

Symptoms/Signs: Hand deformities, short, obese, cardiac abnormalities, low-set hairline, long ear crura, facial asymmetry, midfacial hypoplasia, limb abnormalities, developmental delay, hearing loss

CHIARI MALFORMATIONS[1,4]

Aka Chiari Complex (because they are not isolated entities)

TYPE I

Small posterior fossa with cerebellar tonsil inferior displacement below the foramen magnum 4 (adult)–6 (child) mm

Epidemiology: May present in childhood or as an adult

Associated with: Klippel-Feil, platybasia, suboccipital dysplasia, skull base anomaly (30%), hydromyelia (40%)

Symptoms/Signs: Asymptomatic, headache (tension or exercise induced), lower CN palsies, hydrocephalus, sleep apnea, ataxia, hand weakness, sensory changes, Lhermitte's sign, scoliosis, hydromyelia

TYPE II

Small posterior fossa, large foramen magnum, low torcula heterophili, inferiorly displaced medulla and cerebellum (kinked cervicomedullary junction), beaked tectum (fusion of inferior colliculi), lacunar skull changes (Luckenschadel), tonsil and vermis herniation

Associated with: Myelomeningocele (near 100%), syringomyelia (frequent), colpocephaly, polymicrogyria, agenesis of corpus callosum, hydrocephalus, basilar impression, dysplastic cranial nerve nuclei, absent septum pellucidum

Symptoms/Signs: Downbeat nystagmus, dysphagia, apnea, stridor, upper extremity weakness, lower cranial nerve palsies

TYPE III

Type II + occipital cerebelloencephalocele

TYPE IV

Cerebellar hypoplasia, no encephalocele

DANDY-WALKER MALFORMATION[1,7]

Agenesis of cerebellar vermis with intracerebellar cyst
- Possibly related to 4th ventricle obstruction from atresia of foramina of Luschka and Magendie, superior medullary velum, floor of the 4th ventricle

Associated with: Corpus callosum agenesis, heterotopias, polymicrogria, aqueductal stenosis, hydrocephalus, cephaloceles, polydactyly, spina bifida, Klippel-Feil Syndrome, cleft palate, cardiovascular anomalies

- Outcome is related to the severity of the associated anomalies

Radiology: Large posterior fossa cyst, high insertion of venous torcula, hydrocephalus, agenesis of cerebellar vermis

Symptoms/Signs: Macrocrania, cerebellar dysfunction, papilledema, nystagmus, hydrocephalus, developmental delay

- Some may present only with a delay in walking and may be normal in all other respects

AQUEDUCTAL STENOSIS

Congenital or acquired stenosis of the sylvian aqueduct
- Most cases occur in children, but some present in adulthood
- Acquired cases often due to inflammation (following hemorrhage or infection), tumor (e.g., tectal glioma or pineal region tumor), quadrigeminal plate arachnoid cyst, etc.

Radiology: Characterized by a normal sized 4th ventricle and enlarged 3rd and lateral ventricles on CT or MRI ("triventricular" or noncommunicating hydrocephalus)

Symptoms: Headache, visual change, mental deterioration, gait disturbance, endocrine abnormality, nausea/vomiting, seizures

Signs: Papilledema, intellectual impairment, ataxia, pyramidal tract signs, increased head circumference, full anterior fontanelle

Treatment: Ventriculoperitoneal shunt or endoscopic 3rd ventriculostomy (if > 6 months of age)

NEUROCUTANEOUS SYNDROMES (PHAKOMATOSES)

Also includes VHL, hereditary hemorrhagic telangiectasia, blue rubber bleb nevus syndrome, and Wyburn-Mason syndrome

NEUROFIBROMATOSIS[1]

■ Type 1 (Von Recklinghausen's Disease)

Epidemiology: M = F

Symptoms/Signs and associated findings: Diagnostic criteria must have > 2/7 affected 1st-degree relatives, > six cafe au lait spots, neurofibromas (cranial nerves), axiliary and/or inguinal freckling, optic glioma (pilocytic astrocytomas. Presents with abnormal pupillary light reflex, precocious puberty, Lisch nodules (hamartomas of the iris), distinctive osseous lesions (scoliosis, pseudoarthrosis, sphenoid wing dysplasia)

- Plexiform neurofibromas are pathognomonic
- May also have vascular abnormalities (e.g., MoyaMoya), pulsatile exopthalmos from dysplasia of greater sphenoid wing (orbit, V1, sphenoid wing hypoplasia, middle cranial fossa cyst), orbital globe enlargement, buphthalmos (cow-eye, due to lid neurofibroma), retinal phakomas, plexiform neuromas (V1), visceral and endocrine tumors, intracranial tumors (except acoustic schwannomas; e.g., glioma of brainstem, hypothalamus, 3rd ventricle), macrocephaly, mental retardation, seizures, aqueductal stenosis, pectus excavatus, renal artery stenosis, aneurysms, pheochromocytoma, scoliosis, syrinx
- Spine: Neurofibromas, dural ectasia, arachnoid cysts, acute angle kyphoscoliosis, lateral thoracic meningocele, spinal cord gliomas and hamartomas, enlarged foramen, vertebral scalloping

Genetics: AD (chromosome 17 with gene product neurofibromin, which functions as a tumor suppressor) or sporadic (50% mutation in NF-1 gene, normally inhibits p21-ras), 100% penetrant, variable expressivity

- Neurofibromin: Tumor suppressor, inhibits ras oncogene by inc Ras-GTPase (also EGFR, p53)

Pathology: Myelin vacuolization, dysplastic neurons, microcysts, meningoangiomatosis

■ Type 2 (Bilateral Acoustic Neurofibromatosis)

Genetics: AD, chromosome 22

- Merlin (neurofibromin 2, schwannomin): Links membrane to actin cytoskeleton, tumor suppressor
- Also in non-NF2 schwannomas and meningiomas

Symptoms/Signs and associated findings: Hearing loss, vestibular dysfunction

- Tumors: Bilateral vestibular nerve (acoustic) schwannomas, trigeminal or other cranial nerve schwannomas, ependymoma, meningiomas, astrocytomas
- Skin plaques (NO Lisch nodules or cerebrovascular abnormalities), juvenile cataracts, calcified choroid plexus, normal IQ

TUBEROUS SCLEROSIS (BOURNEVILLE DISEASE)[1,10]

Epidemiology: 1/10,000, M = F

Pathophysiology: Dysfunction of neural migration

Symptoms/Signs and associated findings: Benign tumor (subependymal giant cell astrocytoma) and malformations (hamartoma, aneurysms) of the central nervous system, skin, kidney, heart (50% of all cases of cardiac rhabdomyoma), retina (phakomas/angiomyolipoma), liver (adenoma), pulmonary

- Classic triad of mental retardation (65%), seizures (90%), and adenoma sebaceum (angiofibromas of the face)
- Additional symptoms include autism, hyperactivity, impulsivity, aggression, ash leaf spots, subungal fibromas, shagreen patch
- CNS tumors: Hamartomas (95%), cortical tubers, subependymal nodules, subependymal giant cell astrocytomas (15%)

Genetics: Autosomal dominant

- Chromosome 9 (TSC1, hamartin, gene encodes tumor suppressor), 11, 16 (TSC2, tuberin, gene encodes protein with homology to GAP3 → cell cycle control)
- 80% penetrance, variable expressivity, high spontaneous occurrence rate

Radiology: Hamartomas—hypointense T1, hyperintense T2

- Cortical tubers: < 5% enhance, no transformation, appear like thick gyri
- Subependymal nodules: "Candle gutterings," 30% enhance, calcifications
- Subependymal giant cell astrocytomas: Frequently located at the foramen of Monro, enhance brightly, can obstruct the ventricle causing hydrocephalus

STURGE-WEBER SYNDROME (ENCEPHALOFACIAL ANGIOMATOSIS)

Facial and leptomeningeal angiomatosis

Genetics: Sporadic

Symptoms/Signs and associated findings: V1 port-wine stain, focal seizures, contralateral hemiparesis, hemianesthesia, skull thickening, tram-track calcification of cortex, hemiatrophy of the brain, ipsilateral large enhancing choroid ipsilateral, glaucoma, mental retardation, homonymous hemianopsia, eye angioma

Pathophysiology: Residual embryonal blood vessels

- A vascular plexus in the 6th week around the cephalic portion of the neural tube becomes the facial skin, usually regresses at 9th week of gestation, failure of regression leads to angioma

Radiology: Strong pial enhancement of the angiomas ipsilateral to the facial nevus

Pathology: Multiple thin-walled venules on the parieto-occipital region of the ipsilateral hemisphere to the V1 distribution port-wine stain → chronic ischemia → dystrophic ("tram-track") calcifications and cortical atrophy

- No cortical bridging veins → dilated deep cerebral veins

Treatment: May require hemispherectomy for seizure control

■ Klippel-Trenaunay-Weber Syndrome[11]

Sturge-Weber variant
- Cutaneous and spinal cord hemangiomas found along similar dermatomal distributions
- Classic triad of port-wine stain, varicose veins, and bony and soft-tissue hypertrophy of an extremity

VEIN OF GALEN MALFORMATION[6,12]

Table 7-10 Yasargil Numbering System for Vein of Galen Malformation

1	Few feeders, pericallosal, posterior cerebral • pure fistula of ACA or PCA branch to vein of Galen
2	Fistulous thalamoperforating arteries to vein of Galen
3	Mixed supply*
4	Secondary—shunting of parenchymal or dural plexiform AVM** into normal vein of Galen

* most common
** 1% of all AVM involve the vein of Galen

Table 7-11 Presentation of Vein of Galen Malformation

Age	Presentation
Neonate	High output congestive heart failure, heart murmur, macrocephaly, intracranial bruit
Infant	Seizures, hydrocephalus
Children, Adults	Headache, intracranial hemorrhage

Radiology: Isointense mass posterior to the 3rd ventricle

Treatment: Endovascular (both transarterial and transvenous), observation with management of hydrocephalus, open surgical techniques

Outcome: Depends on age at presentation, cardiac status, and presence of calcifications in the basal ganglia (a marker of cererbral injury due to steal)

GENERAL PEDIATRIC BRAIN TUMOR INFORMATION

Table 7-12 Incidence of Common Pediatric Brain Tumors*

Tumor Type	% of Total
Infratentorial	
Astrocytomas	15
Medulloblastomas	14
Ependymomas	9
Brainstem gliomas	12
Supratentorial	
Astrocytomas WHO grade I (e.g., pilocytic, PXA) & II (e.g., fibrillary, protoplasmic) WHO grade III (anaplastic astrocytoma) & IV (anaplastic glioma or GBM)	13 20
Oligodendrogliomas	2–3
Ependymomas	4
Ganglion cell tumors (gangliogliomas, desmoplastic infantile gangliogliomas, gangliocytomas)	1–7
Embryonal tumors (PNET, AT/RT, neuroblastomas, etc.)	40

*Excludes pineal region tumors
Sources: Albright[13], Greenberg[14]

LOCATION OF PEDIATRIC BRAIN TUMORS

Table 7-13 Location of Pediatric Brain Tumors

Age (months)	Infratentorial (in %)
0–6	27
6–12	53
12–24	74
2–16 years	42

PEDIATRIC HEAD TRAUMA[14]

Epidemiology: 1/500 cases per year

- When compared to adults, children have a lower chance of a surgical lesion in a comatose child

- Pediatric-specific head injuries include birth injuries (e.g., skull fractures, cephalohematoma, leptomeningeal cysts) and nonaccidental trauma (e.g., shaken baby syndrome)

Response to injury: Malignant cerebral edema—occasional sudden onset of cerebral swelling (likely due to hyperemia)

Outcome: Trauma is a leading cause of pediatric deaths

- Pediatric head trauma mortality 28%
- Post-traumatic seizure incidence 1–24 times higher in children

GERMINAL MATRIX HEMORRHAGE (GMH)

Vessels of the germinal matrix in the developing brain are extremely fragile. This, coupled with immature cerebral circulatory autoregulation, puts premature infants at high risk of GMH.

Presentation: Stupor, posturing, seizures, tense fontanelle, apneic and bradycardic spells, loss of pupillary reaction, hematocrit drop > 10%, blood in CSF

- *Hydrocephalus develops in 20–50%.* Grades III and IV GMH have higher risk of progressive hydrocephalus requiring CSF diversion

Risk factors: Asphyxia, volume expansion, seizures, pneumothorax, cyanotic heart disease, mechanical ventilation, ECMO (due to heparinization), maternal cocaine abuse

Epidemiology: 40–45% of preemies < 1500 gm; many GMH asymptomatic

Workup: Ultrasound through fontanelles

- Follow head circumferences daily (91% sensitivity, 85% specificity)

Treatment: Optimize CPP without excessive elevation of CBF. Hydrocephalus can be managed in some via serial LPs. LPs do not reduce likelihood of needing permanent shunting. Ventricular access device (VAD) may be placed to facilitate regular taps, depending on US and OFC trends (20–50% have progressive hydrocephalus). Options beyond VAD include EVD and early shunting.

Insertion of VP shunt: Indicated for symptomatic hydrocephalus, no evidence of infection, CSF protein < 100 mg/dl, infant weight > 2500 gm (or just prior to discharge). Do not tap the reservoir 24 hr prior to VPS placement to allow ventricles to expand pre-op.

Outcomes: Short term—GMH confers higher mortality

- Outcome depends upon birth weight and pulmonary status

Table 7-14 Germinal Matrix Hemorrhage Grading System

Grade	Description
I	Confined to subependyma
II	Interventricular hemorrhage (IVH) without hydrocephalus
III	IVH with hydrocephalus
IV	IVH with parenchymal hemorrhage

CHOROID PLEXUS HEMORRHAGE

Most common cause of interventricular hemorrhage in term neonate
- Symptoms range from asymptomatic to hydrocephalus and increased intracranial pressure

NEURAL TUBE DEFECTS[1,4-6]

Error in primary neurulation
- Decreased incidence with folate supplementation
- Leads to increased levels of alpha-fetoprotein in maternal serum

CRANIORACHISCHISIS

Entire neural tube fails to close → spontaneous abortion

ANENCEPHALY

Epidemiology: F > M

Pathophysiology: Failure of closure of anterior neuropore

Diagnostics: Ultrasound, increased maternal serum alpha-fetoprotein levels

Pathology: Hypoplastic cranial vault with cerebrovasculosa (mass of immature blood vessels) and no brain or only partial brain development (brainstem)

Outcome: Not compatible with survival

ENCEPHALOCELE

Epidemiology: M > F except occipital

Pathophysiology: Herniation of brain tissue through bony skull defects

Location: Occipital (75% in western hemisphere), frontal (75% in far east Asia), parietal, transsphenoidal (associated with sellar anomalies, endocrine dysfunction, agenesis of the corpus callosum), sincipital (southeast Asia)

■ Subtypes and Syndromes

Basal Encephaloceles: Present with CSF leak, recurrent meningitis, nasal mass with airway obstruction

Nasal glioma: Heterotopic lesions not connected to the brain and, therefore, are not true encephaloceles

Meckel-Gruber syndrome: AR

- Occipital encephalocele, hepatic fibrosis, bile duct proliferation, polycystic kidneys
- Outcome is fatal

Meningoencephalocele: Herniation of brain and meningeal tissue through bony skull defects

Hydroencephalomeningocele: Herniation of brain, meninges, and ventricle through bony skull defects

Treatment: Surgical correction unless the amount of herniated brain tissue is greater than the remaining intracranial brain tissue

SPINA BIFIDA OCCULTA[6]

("closed" NTD)

Includes tethered spinal cord, lipomyelomeningocele, lipomeningocele, thickened filum terminale, fatty filum terminale, diastematomyelia, diplomyelia, dermal sinus tract with spinal cord involvement, myelocystocele, anterior sacral meningocele

Defect of posterior vertebral column elements
- No involvement of neural elements or meninges
- May be associated with diastematomyelia, spinal lipoma, spinal dermoid, sinus tract, hyperhidrosis

Symptoms/Signs: Usually asymptomatic

- Cutaneous stigmata (capillary hemangioma, dimple, asymmetric gluteal cleft, subcutaneous lipoma, hypertrichosis, dermal sinus tract)
- May present with symptoms of tethered cord (urologic neurogenic bladder, incontinence, delay in toilet training, scoliosis), orthopedic deformities, sacral agenesis

CHAPTER 8 ■ BRAIN TUMORS[1-5]

Gordon Li, MD

OVERVIEW

Incidence and Outcomes[6]: According to the Central Brain Tumor Registry of the United States, there were an estimated 51,410 new cases of primary nonmalignant and malignant CNS tumors in 2007 (16.5 cases per 100,000 person—years, 9.2 per 100,000 person—years for nonmalignant tumors and 7.3 per 100,000 person—years for malignant tumors); of those, 3,750 were childhood primary CNS tumors. The incidence and mortality rates of these tumors have not changed significantly over the past decade

- Brain tumors remain the leading cause of solid tumor cancer death in the pediatric population and are the second most common cancer in children after leukemia
- There are an estimated 100,000 to 170,000 new cases of brain metastases diagnosed each year in the United States. The most common tumors to metastasize to the brain are lung, breast, melanoma, renal, and colon cancers

Location and Types: Most adult brain tumors are supratentorial. The most common tumor types are brain metastases, gliomas (more common in males), meningiomas (more common in females), sellar region tumors, and vestibular schwannomas. Pediatric brain tumors in children more than 2 years old are more often intratentorial. The most common tumor types are pilocytic astrocytomas, medulloblastomas, brainstem gliomas, and ependymomas. The most common childhood supratentorial tumors are low-grade astrocytomas, craniopharyngiomas, and optic nerve gliomas. CNS tumors in children less than 2 years old, however, are usually supratentorial and are generally highly malignant. The most common CNS tumors in this age group include immature teratomas, central nervous system primitive neuroectodermal tumors (PNET), high-grade astrocytomas, and choroid plexus papillomas/carcinomas.

- Intracranial CNS tumors can be either benign or malignant. Even benign tumors of the CNS can be devastating, however, if they are allowed to grow unchecked within the rigid skull or if they are located in or near a particular critical structure (e.g., a chordoma adjacent to the brainstem). Malignant tumors generally display rapid growth, cellular atypia, and poor differentiation, many mitotic figures, neovascularization, and necrosis
- Long-term follow-up of patients who have undergone brain irradiation shows an increased incidence of both benign and malignant brain tumors.

Genetics: Genetic factors in tumorigenesis include expression of oncogenes, inactivation of tumor suppressor genes, or overexpression of genes of growth factors or their receptors (i.e., EGFR). Only a small percentage of tumors is associated with heritable conditions such as tuberous sclerosis or neurofibromatosis, however

Symptoms: Tend to be insidious and gradually worsen over weeks to months or years. Seizures and acute onset of headache, reflecting, hydrocephalus or intratumoral hemorrhage can lead to acute presentation. Signs and symptoms may result from increased intracranial pressure (from the tumor mass or from CSF obstruction) or direct mass effect on CNS structures (usually resulting in focal neurological deficit). These include but are not limited to headaches, nausea/vomiting, papilledema, seizures, altered mental status, weakness, sensory changes, cranial nerve dysfunction, speech problems, and endocrine dysfunction

Workup: Usually includes CT and MRI scanning and, occasionally, angiography for preoperative embolization of tumor vessels

Treatment: Lesions with surrounding edema are often treated with corticosteroids; patients who present with seizures are treated with antiepileptic therapy. Prophylactic treatment with antiepileptics of a patient with a brain tumor who has not seized is not indicated. Once the diagnosis of a CNS neoplasm is made, then treatment options include serial imaging observation, surgery, radiation therapy, and chemotherapy

GLIAL TUMORS

ASTROCYTOMAS

Epidemiology: Most common primary brain tumor

- Most often between the ages of 40 and 60 years
- M:F = 2:1
- Multifocal in 5% of cases

Grading: I–IV according to World Health Organization (WHO)

- Based on pleomorphism, hypercellularity, vascular proliferation, necrosis
- Grade I = well-circumscribed tumor without nuclear atypia, increased mitoses, anaplasia, necrosis, or neovascularization
- Grade II = nuclear atypia, increased cellularity
- Grade III = increased mitotic index and anaplasia
- Grade IV = nuclear atypia, mitoses, endothelial proliferation, and necrosis (mnemonic "AMEN")

Prognosis: Generally depends on age, histology/grade, Karnofsky score, and extent of resection

■ Grade I Astrocytoma
Generally well circumscribed and usually do not progress to higher grade astrocytomas

- Includes pilocytic astrocytoma, subependymal giant cell astrocytoma (SEGA), and pleomorphic xanthoastrocytoma (PXA)

Pilocytic Astrocytoma

Epidemiology: Account for 1/3 of pediatric gliomas (most common glioma in children)

- 5 to 10% of all gliomas
- Peak incidence around age 10
- 10% of cerebral and 85% of cerebellar astrocytomas
- Optic gliomas common in NF1 patients

Location: Most often cerebellum, followed by brain stem, optic pathway, thalamus, and hypothalamus

Radiology: Often cystic and well circumscribed with a characteristic contrast-enhancing mural nodule, though can be solid

- Usually noncystic in the medulla and optic pathway
- Almost always contrast enhancing

Pathology: Rosenthal fibers (GFAP+), biphasic, microcysts, eosinophilic granular bodies (EGBs), vascular proliferation, microcystic

- Rare necrosis/mitoses

Treatment: Resection of the enhancing nodule and any enhancing cyst wall is indicated

Outcome: Gross total resection usually curative and survival is 86–100% at 5 years, 83% at 10 years, and 70% at 20 years

- Hypothalamic gliomas have a poor prognosis
- If the tumor cannot be totally resected, then survival also worse

Pleomorphic Xanthoastrocytoma (PXA)

Epidemiology: Peak incidence at age 7–25

- Often present with seizures

Location: Superficial temporal lobe

Radiology: Heterogeneous cystic mass with a mural nodule, calcifications

- Often involve the cortex and leptomeninges but not the dura

Treatment: Gross total resection often curative, although some reports of transformation to glioblastoma (GBM)

Pathology: Bizarre pleomorphic astrocytes with xanthomatous fat cells, spindle cells, a rich reticulin network, and no necrosis

Outcome: Favorable prognosis

Subependymal Giant Cell Astrocytoma (SEGA)

Epidemiology: Peak incidence at < 20 years of age

- Often cause hydrocephalus and seizures
- Seen in 15% of tuberous sclerosis (TS) patients

Location: Foramen of Monro

Radiology: Heterogeneous enhancement with frequent calcifications, well circumscribed

Outcome: Tumors benign, but cases of sudden death have been reported from tumor blocking the foramen of Monro and causing a sudden increase in intracranial pressure (ICP)

Pathology: Large multinucleated cells, benign

■ Grade II (Diffuse) Astrocytoma

Subtypes: Protoplasmic, gemistocytic (worse prognosis), fibrillary, or mixed (worse prognosis if > 20% gemistocytes)[7]

Epidemiology: Younger adults with a mean onset of 30 years

Location: White matter

Radiology: Generally diffuse but can be pseudocircumscribed, hypodense on CT, often low on T1 and bright on T2, and generally nonenhancing or minimally enhancing

Outcome: Have a far greater tendency to progress in grade than grade I astrocytomas

- 5-year survival after gross total resection and radiation is 70% but this decreases to 38% with subtotal resection
- Median survival approximately 8.2 years
- Controversial optimal treatment paradigm

Pathology: Unlike in higher grade astrocytomas, mitoses and anaplasia generally absent

- Also lack of necrosis or neovascularization
- Gemistocytic tumors have prominent eosinophilic cytoplasm, peripherally displaced nuclei, and perivascular lymphocytic infiltrate

■ Grade III (Anaplastic) Astrocytoma

Epidemiology: Mean age of presentation in 40s to 50s with slight male predominance

Location: Preference for cerebral hemispheres, but can present almost anywhere in CNS

Radiology: Typically rim enhancing (though many are not) with surrounding vasogenic edema; some have hemorrhage

Pathology: Nuclear atypia, frequent mitoses, increased cellularity, significant proliferative activity, no necrosis or neovascularization

Genetics: High frequency of p53 mutations and LOH 17p

Outcome: Strong tendency to progress to grade IV

- Better outcome for Karnofsky score > 70, age < 45, location amenable to resection, minimal medical comorbidities
- Median survival of patients with anaplastic astrocytomas is 2–3 years

▦ Grade IV (Glioblastoma [GBM]) Astrocytoma

Subset: Gliosarcomas = GBMs with a sarcoma component

Epidemiology: 55% of astrocytomas

- Age 50s to 70s though younger and older patients can present with GBM as well
- GBMs can be primary (i.e., tumors that occur de novo) or secondary (i.e., tumors that start as lower grade astrocytomas and then progress into GBM)

Location: Frontotemporal most common though can present almost anywhere in the CNS

- Occasionally multicentric (3–6%)
- Can invade deep white matter tracts and cross corpus callosum (butterfly glioma)

Radiology: Typically rim enhancing with central necrosis, surrounding vasogenic edema; may hemorrhage

- ~4% do not enhance with contrast

Pathology: Nuclear atypia, frequent mitoses, endothelial proliferation, necrosis, secondary structures of Scherer (tumor cells surrounding neurons in the gray matter or infiltrating along white matter tracts), pseudopallisading necrosis, and glomeruloid vascular proliferation

Genetics: Primary pathway tumors more often have mutations of the EGF receptor and loss of PTEN while secondary pathway tumors more often have p53 mutations

Outcome: Poor

- Better outcome for Karnofsky score > 70, age < 45, location amenable to resection, minimal medical comorbidities
- Median survival of patients who receive current standard of care including resection, postoperative radiation, and temozolomide = 12–15 months
- GBM survival without treatment = 3–6 months
- Primary and secondary pathway tumors have same prognosis

Gliomatosis Cerebri:

Diffusely infiltrating glioma involving at least three lobes at diagnosis (can be bilateral) with minimal mass effect

- Largely nonenhancing, though some areas can show mild enhancement
- Can often present differently from other high grade gliomas (cognitive/behavioral symptoms or other ill-defined neurologic deficits)
- Poor prognosis

■ Brainstem Glioma

Epidemiology: 10–20% of pediatric brain tumors

- Often present with cranial nerve palsies and headache
- Heterogeneous group of tumors, but 58–75% are diffuse infiltrating
- Other types include tectal gliomas, focal brainstem gliomas, and cervicomedullary gliomas

Location: Midbrain, pons, medulla

Radiology: Diffuse-intrinsic brainstem glioma is an infiltrative lesion that often results in marked brainstem enlargement

- Hyperintense on T2
- Variable enhancement

Pathology: Diffuse-infiltrating glioma is a grade II to IV astrocytoma

- Focal brainstem glioma, tectal glioma, and cervicomedullary gliomas are usually low-grade astrocytomas

Treatment: Radiation therapy for diffuse-infiltrating type

- No surgery for diffuse type, though focal lesions can be removed safely
- Tectal gliomas (limited to tectum, generally nonenhancing) often need only CSF diversion (3rd ventriculostomy or ventriculoperitoneal shunt)

Outcome: Diffuse type is progressive and fatal

- Well-circumscribed grade 1 lesions and tectal gliomas have an excellent prognosis
- CSF diversion may be considered for palliation of obstructive hydrocephalus

OLIGODENDROGLIOMA

Epidemiology: Typically found in adults (rarely in children)

- Peak age 35 to 40 years
- Often present with seizures

Location: Generally frontotemporal lobes though can present almost anywhere

Radiology: Have a higher frequency of hemorrhaging

- Often contain irregular calcifications
- Mild heterogeneous enhancement with contrast

Pathology: Classic fried-egg appearance (an artifact of permanent sections but not frozen sections), round nuclei, "chicken-wire" vasculature, perineuronal satellitosis, calcifications, intratumoral hemorrhage, and pseudocysts

- Grade II lesions have marked nuclear atypia and occasional mitosis while grade III (anaplastic) lesions have significant mitotic activity, prominent microvascular proliferation, or necrosis

Genetics: Subset has codeletion of 1p and 19q, which correlates with sensitivity to treatment and improved prognosis

Outcome: 5-year survival 75%

- Better prognosis than astrocytomas or mixed oligoastrocytomas (especially with 1p/19q deletion) with median survival times of 11.6 years for grade II and 3.5 years for grade III

EPENDYMOMA

Subtypes: Pathologic variants include cellular, papillary, epithelial, clear cell, mixed, tanycytic, myxopapillary (grade I)

- Grade II or grade III (anaplastic)

Epidemiology: Constitute 5% of adult intracranial gliomas, 10% of childhood CNS tumors

- Associated with neurofibromatosis 2 (often multiple)
- Bimodal peak of occurrence at ages 1 to 5 and age 35
- M = F

Location: From the lining of ventricles or central canal of spinal cord

- Generally intracranial in children and spinal (60% of intramedullary spinal cord tumors, most often at the filum) or less commonly, ventricular in adults
- Typically centered in the 4th ventricle and extend through the foramina of Luschka and Magendie
- In spinal cord, often associated with a syrinx, which creates a good margin for resection (versus spinal cord astrocytomas, which do not have a good resection margin)

Radiology: Isointense on T1, intermediate to mildly hyperintense on T2

- Well circumscribed
- Enhance with contrast
- Spinal cord lesions may be associated with cysts, syrinx formation, and hemosiderin deposition

Pathology: Ependymomas have classic true rosette (polygonal tumor cells around a central canal) or perivascular pseudorosettes (polygonal tumor cells around a blood vessel)

- Cysts
- Surface microvilli
- Mitotic figures (grade III)
- +GFAP, +EMA

Location: Varied, depends on age, location, and grade

- E.g., most childhood ependymomas present in the 4th ventricle while myxopapillary ependymomas usually occur along the filum terminale
- In children less than 2 years of age, ependymomas are commonly supratentorial

Outcome: Supratentorial ependymomas in young children have worse prognosis than posterior fossa ependymoma in older children

- Gross total resection improves overall survival
- Better prognosis for > 3 yrs old
- Need to obtain full craniospinal MRI to evaluate for CSF spread, which has a worse prognosis

■ Myxopapillary Ependymoma

Grade 1

- Commonly associated with the conus medullaris or filum terminale
- Isointense on T1, iso-to hyperintense on T2; contrast enhancing
- On path, ependymocytes arranged around papillary projections containing myxoid stroma
- Can be cured with gross total resection, unless it invades the conus

SUBEPENDYMOMA

Epidemiology: Rare

- Peak age of 40 to 60 years
- M > F

Pathology: Grade I, benign

- 50% of symptoms because of CSF obstruction

Location: 4th ventricle, body of lateral ventricle or sometimes in the spinal cord

Radiology: Often nonenhancing (whereas most intraventricular tumors enhance)

- Well circumscribed
- Mild hyperintensity on T2

Pathology: Both ependymal and astrocytic features

- Grouped nodular cells

Treatment: Cured with gross total resection

Asymptomatic lesions can be followed

CHOROID PLEXUS PAPILLOMA (CPP)

Epidemiology: Peak age of less than 10 years (85% before age 5, most even before age 2, especially when in the lateral/3rd ventricles)

- Benign, slow growing
- Often present with hydrocephalus due to obstruction and/or increased CSF production

Outcome: Good after resection because they rarely transform to a more aggressive histology (choroid plexus carcinoma), but these tumors can recur and disseminate through the CSF

Location: Intraventricular (commonly in the atrium of the left ventricle in children and in the 4th ventricle in adults)

Radiology: Multilobulated "cauliflower" morphology

- Enhance intensely after contrast infusion

Pathology: Neoplasm of the epithelial cells of the choroid plexus

- Closely resembles normal choroid plexus except more crowded
- Increased mitotic activity alone connotes atypical choroid plexus papilloma
- Tumors with at least four of the following five features (Frequent mitoses, increased cellular density, nuclear pleomorphism) blurring of the papillary pattern with poorly structured sheets of tumor cells, and necrosis are WHO grade III choroid plexus carcinomas (accounts for 15% of CP tumors)
- Choroid plexus carcinoma typically invades brain parenchyma and causes edema

NEURONAL AND MIXED NEUROGLIAL TUMORS

GANGLIOGLIOMA

Epidemiology: 1% of CNS tumors

- Most commonly present in the first 3 decades (80% < 30 years)
- Slowly growing
- Typically present with seizures

Pathology: Contain both neuronal and glial components

- Dysmorphic, binucleate ganglion ("owl eyes")
- Anaplastic ganglioglioma has malignant features
- + synaptophysin, neurofilament MAPII, GFAP
- A subset have neuronal but not glial components

Location: Peripheral cortical location

- Predilection for the temporal lobes > parietal >> cerebellum

Radiology: May be solid or mixed cystic and solid (~50%)

- Mass effect depends on size; often little or no edema
- Calcifications frequent (~50%)
- Enhancement is variable

Treatment: Surgical resection

DYSPLASTIC GANGLIOCYTOMA OF THE CEREBELLUM (LHERMITTE-DUCLOS DISEASE)

Epidemiology: Rare

- Associated with Cowden syndrome (multisystem disease involving hamartomatous overgrowth of tissue and increased risk of thyroid, breast, and other cancers; most cases with germ-line PTEN mutation)

- Slowly progressive, variably associated with cerebellar signs and symptoms of raised intracranial pressure

Radiology: Focal region of cerebellar folia thickening and fissural effacement

- Hypointense on T1, alternating "stripes" on T2, nonenhancing

Pathology: Diffuse enlargement of the internal granular layers of the cerebellum, which are filled by ganglionic cells, with preservation of the cerebellar architecture

Treatment: Decompression of the posterior fossa by total surgical removal of the mass

DESMOPLASTIC INFANTILE GANGLIOGLIOMA (DIG)

Epidemiology: Rare

- First 18 months of life
- WHO grade 1

Location: Supratentorial tumor

- Usually frontal or parietal lobe
- Involves overlying dura

Radiology: Both solid and cystic components

- Solid component usually peripheral, enhancing
- Cystic portion more medial, often massive

Treatment: Surgical resection

Prognosis: Generally curable with gross total resection

DYSEMBRYOPLASTIC NEUROEPITHELIAL TUMORS (DNET)

Epidemiology: Young adults and children

- Present with seizures

Location: Supratentorial (predilection for temporal lobes)

Pathology: Contain mixed neural and glial elements and have an association with cortical dysplasia

- Thought to arise from the external granular layer of the cortex
- Floating neurons on loose background with big microcysts
- Multinodular

Radiology: Cortically based lesion; usually no edema, minimal mass effect

- Often small cysts
- Variable nodular enhancement

Treatment: Surgical resection usually curative

CENTRAL NEUROCYTOMA

Epidemiology: Young adults

Location: Within the lateral ventricles at septum pellucidum or foramen of Monro

Pathology: Grade II

- Neuronal in origin
- Do not infiltrate
- Uniform cells on "ground glass" neuropil background
- + synaptophysin

Radiology: Well-circumscribed, lobulated lateral ventricular mass

- Heterogeneous, "feathery" enhancement
- Frequently have punctate calcifications, small cysts

Treatment: Gross total resection usually curative

- Radiation is effective for growing residual or recurrent tumor

PINEAL TUMORS

Symptoms: Classic presentation is Parinaud syndrome—upward gaze palsy, pupillary dilation, lid retraction, nystagmus, and light-near dissociation

Pineal parenchymal tumors make up ~20% of pineal region tumors

PINEOCYTOMA

A well-circumscribed, slowly growing, and well-differentiated tumor with peak incidence of 30 years
- Associated cysts are common

PINEOBLASTOMAS

Related to central nervous system primitive neuroectodermal tumor or PNETs
- Highly aggressive with poor prognosis
- More common in children
- Pathologic examination reveals small round blue cells with high cellularity and mitoses
- Enhance heterogeneously with contrast, often disseminate through CSF
- May be associated with bilateral retinoblastoma (trilateral retinoblastoma)

TRILATERAL RETINOBLASTOMA

Connotes bilateral retinoblastomas and a pineoblastoma

PINEAL PARENCHYMAL TUMORS OF INTERMEDIATE DIFFERENTIATION

Tumors intermediate between the more benign pineocytoma and the more aggressive pineoblastoma

PAPILLARY TUMORS OF THE PINEAL REGION

Rare pineal parenchymal tumors characterized by papillary architecture and epithelial cytology

EMBRYONAL TUMORS

CENTRAL NERVOUS SYSTEM PRIMITIVE NEUROECTODERMAL TUMOR (PNET)

■ Subtypes

Medulloepithelioma (the most primitive of the PNETs; affects very young children), retinoblastoma (most common extracranial malignant solid tumor in children; derived from neural crest precursor of the sympathetic ganglia; pathogenesis related to loss of tumor suppressor gene RB on chromosome 13), ependymoblastoma, pineoblastoma

MEDULLOBLASTOMA[8]

■ Subtypes

Desmoplastic, medulloblastoma with extensive nodularity, anaplastic, and large cell medulloblastoma

Presentation: Often secondary to hydrocephalus and increased intracranial pressure (headaches, nausea, and vomiting) or cerebellar signs (ataxia, incoordination)

Epidemiology: Most common subtype of PNET

- Most often occur before the age of 10 with a second peak at late 20s
- Male predominance
- 20% of CNS tumors in children
- Most common malignant brain tumor of childhood
- Associated with Gorlin syndrome (aka basal cell nevus syndrome), an autosomal dominant disease related to mutation of PTCH1 gene

Location: Arise from medullary velum, typically fill 4th ventricle

- Occur in the midline in children but more frequently off midline in adults

Genetics: 17q, sonic hedgehog signaling pathway activation, Wnt/wingless signaling activation, TP53 tumor suppressor deficit, MYC oncogene family amplification

Pathology: Embryonal neuroepithelial, originating from external granule layer of cerebellum

- Densely packed cells with round- to oval-shaped hyperchromatic nuclei
- About 40% of the cases have Homer Wright rosettes (a circular or spherical grouping of tumor cells around a pale, eosinophilic, central area that contains neurofibrils but lacks a lumen)
- Desmoplastic synaptophysin islands

Radiology: Mass lesion of the 4th ventricle in young children, cerebellar hemisphere in teenagers and adults

- Hyperdense on CT due to high cellularity and variable calcification
- Typically isointense on T1 and T2

- May contain cysts
- Mild to moderate contrast enhancement
- Often seeds via CSF and full neuraxis MRI is required for staging

Treatment: Surgical resection with postoperative craniospinal radiation and chemotherapy

Prognosis: With standard therapy, 5-year survival approaches 70%

- Medulloblastoma with nodularity type → improved prognosis, anaplastic type → worsened prognosis

ATYPICAL TERATOID/RHABDOID TUMORS (AT/RT)

Presentation: Variable depending on the location (infra- versus supratentorial) of the tumor or age of the patient

- Infants often present with lethargy or nausea and vomiting
- Other signs include head tilt and cranial nerve palsy
- Older children can complain of headaches or weakness

Epidemiology: Children less than age 3

- Rarely seen in children older than 6

Location: Supratentorial lesions slightly more common than infratentorial lesions

- Rarely seen in the spine
- Usually in the cerebellar hemispheres when supratentorial and cerebellar hemispheres, cerebellopontine angle, or brainstem when infratentorial

Radiology: Tumors often large with associated edema

- Imaging characteristics similar to PNET/medulloblastomas
- Seeding of the CSF is common and full neural axis imaging required during workup

Pathology: Combination of rhabdoid, primitive neuroepithelial, epithelial, and mesenchymal components

Genetics: Inactivation of the INI1/hSNF5 gene and the diagnosis can be made with immunohistochemistry showing loss of nuclear INI (i.e., does not stain with INI)

- INI protein is a component of the mammalian SWI/SNF complex that functions in an ATP-dependent manner to alter chromatin structure (the specific role for INI in AT/RT is unknown but thought to be in part due to p16 and p53 pathways)
- Check for rhabdoid tumor predisposition syndrome, a disorder with increased risk of developing malignant rhabdoid tumors due to inactivation or loss of the one allele of the INI gene

Prognosis: Poorest prognosis of the embryonal tumors with overall survival of 1–2 years

TUMORS OF THE CRANIAL AND PARASPINAL/PERIPHERAL NERVES

SCHWANNOMA

Epidemiology: Account for 7% of all intracranial tumors, 80% of cerebellopontine masses (vestibular schwannoma)

- Associated with neurofibromatosis type 2 (NF2) where they are multiple
- Cause neurologic deficit from direct compression
- M = F
- Usual age of presentation 40 to 50 in sporadic cases (20s with NF2 patients)
- Symptoms vary with location: In vestibular schwannoma, sensorineural hearing loss (higher frequencies first), tinnitus, headache, disequilibrium, rarely with facial nerve palsy

Location: Most commonly arise from superior vestibular nerve (vestibular schwannoma aka acoustic neuroma), bilateral in NF2

- Trigeminal nerve
- Other cranial nerves, spinal nerves

Radiology: Round or oval, well-circumscribed masses

- Isointense on T1 weighted imaging, T2 bright, and enhancing
- May have areas of cyst formation, hemorrhage

Pathology: Cytologically benign

- Rarely undergo malignant transformation
- Grossly firm and encapsulated
- Biphasic pattern of Antoni A (compact fusiform spindle cells, reticulin, and collagen) and Antoni B fibers (loosely arranged stellate round cells in stroma)
- Verocay bodies: Groups of spindle cells that look like schools of fish swimming in different directions
- Contain no axons
- S-100+

Treatment: Serial imaging in an asymptomatic patient with small tumor and no brainstem or other critical structure compression

- Enlarging tumors or symptomatic lesions treated with surgery or radiosurgery

Specific for treatment of vestibular schwannoma: Radiosurgery often considered for vestibular schwannoma, especially for smaller tumors without brainstem compression in the elderly or in patients in poor medical condition; rates of hearing loss and facial weakness are less with radiosurgical treatment than with open surgical resection

- Surgical approaches to cerebellopontine angle (CPA) vestibular schwannomas include translabyrinthine (for patients with poor hearing, retrosigmoid, middle fossa-subtemporal

- Complications of CPA surgery include cranial nerve deficits (risk reflects size of tumor), CSF leak, hemorrhage, stroke

MALIGNANT PERIPHERAL NERVE SHEATH TUMOR[9]

Epidemiology: Age 20–50

- 10% of all soft-tissue sarcomas
- 4% of patients with neurofibromatosis I (half of all MPNST diagnoses)
- Painful

Location: Usually in lower extremities, but ~10% are in head/neck, associated with cranial nerves (trigeminal)

Pathology: Dense hypercellular tumor with anaplastic features (schwannoma-like)

Radiology: Look similar to schwannoma, but with a much more rapid growth rate

- May invade adjacent structures, incite brain edema

Treatment: Wide margin surgery

- Adjuvant chemo (high-dose doxorubicin) and usually radiation therapy

Outcome: 75% recur

- 5-year mortality of 50–75%

MENINGEAL TUMORS

MENINGIOMA

■ WHO Grading/Subtypes

- Grade 1: meningothelial, fibrous, transitional, psammomatous, angiomatous, myxoid, secretory (cea +); grade II: chordoid, clear cell; grade III: papillary, rhabdoid, anaplastic

Epidemiology: 15–20% of all intracranial tumors and autopsy studies estimate an incidence of 30%

- 80% of meningiomas are grade 1, 5–20% grade II, and 1–2% grade III
- F > M (especially when in the spine)
- Often express hormonal receptors (progesterone, estrogen, and androgen)
- Patients with meningiomas have a higher incidence of breast cancer and vice versa
- Increased incidence in neurofibromatosis 2
- Multiple in 8%

Genetics: Most commonly, loss of the neurofibromatosis 2 gene on chromosome 22q which encodes a tumor suppressor called merlin (also known as schwannomin)

Location: Typically extra-axial and dural-based, but may arise from choroid plexus in trigone of lateral ventricle; may involve convexity dura, falx, tentorium, dura overlying the skull base, or optic sheath

Radiology: Extra-axial mass (separated from brain by cerebrospinal fluid/vascular cleft)

- Well circumscribed, isointense to brain on T1 and T2 weighted imaging, intense contrast enhancement
- Other characteristic findings include a dural tail (dural enhancement extending away from the primary mass) and hyperostosis of adjacent bone
- Variable calcification
- Rare cystic change or hemorrhage

Pathology: WHO I tumors are benign tumors

- Originate from arachnoid cap cells
- +EMA and vimentin stain
- Wide variety of histologic appearances depending on subtype of meningioma
- Atypical meningiomas have increased mitotic activity (four or more mitoses per 10 high-powered fields) or three or more of the following characteristics: Increased cellularity, small cells with high nuclear to cytoplasmic ratio, prominent nucleoli, uninterrupted patternless or sheet-like growth, and foci of necrosis
- Malignant meningiomas display cytology resembling carcinoma, melanoma, or high-grade sarcoma or have > 20 mitoses per high-powered field

Treatment: Gross total resection is the goal and is generally curative for benign meningiomas

- Radiation (radiosurgery for small tumors) often indicated for poor surgical candidates, subtotal resection, unresectable tumors, or high-grade and recurrent tumors

Prognosis: WHO grade I meningiomas have a greater than 80% chance of progression-free survival at 10 years, while only 40–60% of WHO grade II patients are progression free at 10 years

- Median recurrence-free rate of patients with malignant meningioma is 2 years
- Extent of resection predicts risk of recurrence

HEMANGIOPERICYTOMA

Used to be considered a subtype of meningioma, but now considered a distinct pathologic entity

Epidemiology: M > F

- Mean age of 40 to 50 years

Location: Dural based, supratentorial

Pathology: Staghorn vascular channels and absence of the whorls or psammoma bodies seen in meningiomas

- Pericyte cell is postulated to be the cell of origin

Treatment: Endovascular embolization followed by surgery

- Tumor does not respond well to radiation or chemotherapy

Prognosis: Recurrence rates approximately 70% even with gross total resection

- 5-, 10-, 15-year survival rates are 63%, 37%, 21% respectively
- 10–30% metastasize, especially to lung and bone

MESENCHYMAL TUMORS

HEMANGIOBLASTOMA

Epidemiology: 2% of intracranial tumors and 10% of posterior fossa tumors

- Most common primary posterior fossa brain tumor of adults
- Present with a mean age between 20 to 40 years of age
- M > F
- 80% of these tumors are sporadic and 20% occur in patients with Von Hippel-Lindau syndrome (VHL)
- Secrete erythropoietin → polycythemia

Location: Cerebellar hemispheres > spinal cord > brainstem

- Retina involved in VHL

Radiology: Classically a cystic lesion with an intensely enhancing mural nodule

- 40% can be solid
- Hypervascular and a prominent feeding vessel may be identified
- Often multiple in VHL
- In the spine, often associated with hydromyelia and cord edema

Treatment: Surgical resection versus radiosurgery versus observation depending on size, number, lesion, neurologic deficit, and whether spontaneous lesion or assoicated with VHL; the cyst requires neither resection nor radiation

Outcome: Usually cured with surgery

- Low recurrence rate after gross total resection
- Radiosurgery also has good tumor control rates
- Patients with VHL often have new and multiple lesions despite treatment

CHORDOMA

Epidemiology: < 1% CNS tumors

- Often present with HA, CNVI palsy

Location: Sacrum (50%) > clivus (30%) >> vertebral bodies (usually cervical or upper thoracic)

Radiology: CT shows lytic lesion centered in bone

- Lesion often hypodense on CT
- On MR, hypointense on T1, hyperintense on T2, variable enhancement
- Not usually calcified, but fragments of residual destroyed bone may be present

Pathology: Notochord remnant

- Lobulated, gray, soft with sheets of cords of large vacuolated cells (characteristic physaliferous cells) surrounded by mucin

Treatment: Surgery and high-dose radiation therapy (proton beam, IMRT, and/or radiosurgery)

Outcome: Slowly growing but locally aggressive and invasive

- Depends on extent of resection (complete excision often difficult, especially at skull base)
- 5-year survival 51%, 10-year 35%
- Chordomas metastasize approximately 25–40% and may change to sarcoma
- Recur locally, sometimes along surgical tract

CHONDROSARCOMA

■ Subtypes

Conventional, clear cell, mesenchymal, and dedifferentiated (conventional most common in skull base)

Epidemiology: Second most frequent primary malignant tumor of bone (25% of all primary osseous neoplasms)

- Usually patients > 40 years of age
- M > F

Location: Skull base location most common: petroclival fissure, parasellar, cerebellopontine angle, paranasal sinuses

Radiology: Rounded mass classically located off-midline in the skull base

- Isointense on T1, bright on T2, brightly enhancing postcontrast
- Variable amount of matrix calcification

Pathology: Negative for epithelial membrane antigen (positive in meningioma), positive for S100

- Biphasic pattern of spindle chondroid cells and well-differentiated cartilage in dense fibromyxoid stroma

Treatment: Surgical resection; IMRT or radiotherapy to residual tumor

Outcome: Better prognosis than chordoma with less metastatic potential

INTRACRANIAL LIPOMA

Epidemiology: 0.1% intracranial tumors

- Usually asymptomatic
- Due to persistence of meninx primitiva, so developmental, not neoplastic
- Associated with other congenital abnormalities including callosal dysgenesis, cephaloceles

Location: 30% near corpus callosum

- Also quadrigeminal cistern, tuber cinereum, cerebellopontine angle, internal auditory canal

Radiology: Follows fat on all sequences: hyperintense on T1

- Suppresses on fat-saturation sequences
- May see associated calcifications (osteolipoma)

Pathology: Persistence of meninx primativa (← neural crest)

- Microscopically resemble adipose tissue

Treatment: Usually observed as they are associated with neural structures and normal blood vessels

- Surgery reserved for lesions causing significant mass effect on adjacent structures which is extremely uncommon

LYMPHOMA

Epidemiology: Primary CNS lymphoma (PCNSL) has increased worldwide recently to about 6.6% of all primary intracranial neoplasms because of the AIDS epidemic

- Often seen in immunocompromised patients (i.e., AIDS patients, post-transplant patients or inherited immune disorders such as Wiskott-Aldrich syndrome)
- Epstein-Barr virus (EBV) present in > 95% of tumor cells in PCNSL from immunocompromised patients
- PCNSL affects patients of all ages with a peak incidence in immunocompetent patients during the 6th and 7th decades but younger in immunocompromised patients (10 years for inherited immune patients, 37 years for post-transplant patients, and 39 years for AIDS patients)
- M:F = 3:2

Location: Primary CNS lymphoma usually leads to parenchymal supratentorial masses

- Lesions often multiple
- May involve basal ganglia, corpus callosum, periventricular regions of brain
- Secondary CNS lymphoma (that has spread to CNS from another site in the body) may involve dura or leptomeninges in addition to parenchyma

Radiology: Masses often relatively dense on unenhanced CT due to high cellularity

- Usually intermediate on T1, T2 weighted MR images
- Typically homogeneous enhancement in non–AIDS–related PCNSL, ring-enhancement in AIDS–related PCNSL
- May see mild or moderate reduced diffusion due to high cellularity

Pathology: Perivascular lymphoid cells (B-cell)

Treatment: Biopsy for diagnosis

- Treat with radiation, chemotherapy
- Autologous stem cell transplantation for younger patients is an option

Prognosis: Patients often develop long-term neurotoxicity secondary to combined systemic and intraventricular chemotherapy with whole brain radiation

- Median overall survival is 50 months
- Better in patients less than 61 years of age (75% 5-year survival)

GERM CELL TUMORS (GCT)

Epidemiology: Account for approximately 3% of pediatric brain tumors

- Mean age of 10–20 years (at the onset of puberty in males)

Location: Suprasellar and pineal region

Pathology: Arise from aberrant migration of primordial germ cells

■ Tumor Markers
See Table 8-1

Table 8-1 Germ Cell Tumor Type and Markers

Tumor Type	beta-HCG[a]	AFP[b]	PLAP[c]	c-Kit
Pure Germinoma	-	-	+/-	+
Germinoma (syncytiotrophoblastic)	+	-	+/-	+
Endodermal sinus tumor	-	+	+/-	-
Choriocarcinoma	+	-	+/-	-
Embryonal carcinoma	-	+	+	-
Mixed GCT[d]	+/-	+/-	+/-	+/-
Mature teratoma	-	-	-	-
Immature teratoma	+/-	+/-	-	+/-

[a]beta-HCG: beta-human chorionic gonadotropin
[b]AFP: alpha-fetoprotein
[c]PLAP: placental alkaline phosphatase
[d]GCT: germ cell tumor
Source: Louis D[5]

GERMINOMA

Epidemiology: Most common pineal region tumor (2/3s of the GCTs)

- 1% of all CNS malignancies
- Peak age 10–30 years
- Male predominance (especially Asian)
- Associated with precocious puberty (if sellar/suprasellar)
- Presents with diabetes insipidus (if involves the pituitary stalk/hypothalamus)

Location: Pineal, suprasellar/sellar

- 10% occur both in the pineal and sellar regions
- May also occur in basal ganglia (especially in Asians)

Pathology: Large polygonal cells

- Lack necrosis and hemorrhage
- Infiltration of T-cells

Genetics: Approximately 90% of germ cell tumors are associated with structural chromosomal anomalies, especially an isochromosome on chromosome arm 12p known as i(12p)

- Most germinomas contain c-kit mutations

Laboratory analysis: Alpha-fetoprotein, beta HCG, CSF cytology (see Table 8-1)

Radiology: Hyperdense on CT due to increased cellularity

- Isointense on T1 and T2, homogenously enhancing
- Pituitary stalk involvement may be subtle, so check carefully in young patient presenting with diabetes insipidus
- Full neural axis imaging required because CSF seeding is common

Treatment: Pure germinomas are sensitive to radiation

- Mixed tumor types and other GCTs respond much more poorly to radiation
- Chemotherapy includes cisplatin, etoposide, bleomycin

Outcome: Survival 90% at 10 years

- Recurrence 30%

CHORIOCARCINOMAS

Can be primary or metastatic, usually from testicle
- Prognosis poor
- Propensity to hemorrhage

TERATOMAS

Congenital tumors that can be mature (good prognosis if resectable) or immature (poor prognosis)
- Second most common GCT and usually affects young males

- Contains elements from all three layers (endoderm, mesoderm, and ectoderm) including skin, nerve, cartilage, bone fat, muscle, respiratory glands, and GI glands

SELLAR TUMORS

PITUITARY ADENOMA

Referred to as microadenomas when ≤ 1 cm (75%) and macroadenomas when > 1 cm

- May be functional (hormone secreting) or nonfunctional
- Clinical evaluation should include complete endocrinologic workup and formal visual fields exam (for macroadenomas)

Epidemiology: 10% of intracranial tumors

- Increased incidence in multiple endocrine neoplasia 1 (MEN1)
- F > M with prolactin and ACTH-secreting tumors, M > F with growth hormone–secreting tumors
- If large, may present with bitemporal hemianopsia from compression of the optic chiasm
- Prolactinomas are the most common pituitary tumor

Radiology: CT is not the study of choice, but larger tumors may be seen as isodense sellar/suprasellar mass

- Pituitary apoplexy may cause enlarged hyperdense gland on CT
- Usually intermediate signal intensity on T1 and T2 weighted MRI images
- Enhance moderately, but often less than the normal gland
- Macroadenomas may show cystic or hemorrhagic change
- Sella typically enlarged with macroadenoma

Treatment: Surgery for functioning adenomas secreting TSH, GH, ACTH, or for prolactinomas with visual symptoms or that have failed medical treatment

- Medical therapy for prolactinomas otherwise (see following)

Complications of transsphenoidal surgery: CSF leak, injury to the internal carotid artery, stroke, diabetes insipidus, panhypopituitarism, hemorrhage, sinusitis

■ Prolactinoma

Lactotrophic, acidophilic is the most common pituitary adenoma (30%)

- Can cause amenorrhea and galactorrhea in females and impotence or decreased libido in males (females tend to present earlier due to these symptoms and prolactinomas tend to be larger in males when detected)
- Prolactin level is normally > 150 in patients with these tumors and prolactin level is proportional to the tumor size
- When the prolactin level is elevated but less than 100, this is likely secondary to *stalk effect* rather than a prolactinoma (decreased dopamine

causing increased prolactin from compression of the pituitary stalk by a mass)
- Sometimes large prolactinomas can have spuriously normal prolactin levels (*hook effect*) because the overabundance of prolactin over saturates the lab → 1:100 dilution of the serum sample prior to analysis will clarify the prolactin level in these cases
- These tumors often respond to dopamine agonists (bromocriptine, cabergoline)
- Surgery reserved for medical failure or intolerance of medications

Growth Hormone–Secreting Tumors
Somatotrophic, acidophilic
- Second most common secreting pituitary adenoma (13%)
- Causes acromegaly in adults and gigantism in children
- Treatment is with surgery and octreotide (a somatostatin analog)

Corticotrophic (ACTH)–Secreting Tumors
Basophilic
- Causes Cushing's disease and accounts for 10% of pituitary adenomas
- 40% exhibit *gsp* oncogene mutation

Nelson's Syndrome
Occurs after bilateral adrenalectomy
- Eliminates adrenal cortisol production, therefore releasing the cortisol's negative feedback, which can allow any preexisting pituitary adenoma to grow unchecked
- Continued growth can cause mass effect due to physical compression of brain tissue, along with increased production of ACTH and MSH (causes hyperpigmentation)
- Treatment is surgical

FSH/LH–Secreting Tumors
Account for 9% of pituitary adenomas and generally occur in the elderly

Thyrotrophic or TSH–Secreting Tumors
Basophilic
- Cause hyperthyroidism
- Account for 1% of pituitary adenomas

Nonsecreting Null Cell Tumor (Oncocytoma)
Do not secrete hormone

Pituitary Carcinomas
Rare and display increased mitotic activity, nuclear atypia, and necrosis

Pituitary Apoplexy
Sudden onset of headache with neurological or endocrinologic disturbance due to hemorrhagic necrosis of the pituitary adenoma

Symptoms/Signs: Visual changes, marked endocrine dysfunction (can lead to cardiovascular collapse), ophthalmoplegia, headache

Treatment: Emergent surgery and steroid replacement

CRANIOPHARYNGIOMA

Location: Classically suprasellar mass

Epidemiology: 9% of all pediatric intracranial tumors and 2–5% of all intracranial tumors

- Peak age 0 to 20 years with a second peak at 50 years
- May cause growth retardation, headache, nausea/vomiting, diabetes insipidus, hydrocephalus (3rd ventricle compression), visual field deficits, endocrine dysfunction

Pathology: Derived from squamous cells in Rathke's cleft

- Adamantinomatous (children; cystic with calcifications), papillary (adults; solid without calcification)
- Macroscopically filled with cholesterol-rich fluid with a "motor oil" appearance

Radiology: Macrocysts and calcifications common

- Cysts often bright on T1 due to proteinaceous, hemorrhagic cyst contents
- Heterogeneous enhancement: Rim enhancement around cysts, as well as areas of solid enhancement

Treatment: Surgical resection

- Often recurs especially with subtotal resection or with tumors greater than 5 cm
- Sometimes irradiated
- Can place catheter into the cyst and drain the cyst (can also inject p32 into the cyst for intratumoral treatment)

Outcome: Slowly growing benign tumors, but can invade critical structures causing vision loss, endocrine dysfunction

- Papillary variant (more common in adults) has a better prognosis

RATHKE'S CLEFT CYST

Epidemiology: F > M

- 30 to 40 years old
- May be incidentally found or may present with visual or endocrine (stalk effect) symptoms

Location: Up to 70% both intra- and suprasellar

- May be pre- or retrochiasmatic

Radiology: Cystic lesion that is hypointense on CT, hyperintense on T2

- No calcifications or enhancement

Pathology: Remnant of the craniopharyngeal duct (Rathke's pouch)

- Develops when the proximal part of pars intermedia closes early (day 24) and the distal cleft remains open between the pars distalis and pars nervosa
- Contain watery, mucous fluid lined with ciliated cells and columnar/cuboidal epithelial cells

Treatment: Transsphenoidal surgery if symptomatic

LYMPHOCYTIC HYPOPHYSITIS[10]

Autoimmune inflammatory lesion of pituitary gland

Epidemiology: Young women in late pregnancy or postpartum

Symptoms: Include hyperprolactinemia, headache, visual field deficits, pituitary insufficiency (ACTH earliest and most frequent)

Radiology: Diffuse homogeneous enlargement and enhancement of pituitary gland

- Optic chiasm may be displaced
- May involve surrounding dura → dural tail

Treatment: Steroids

Pathology: Lymphocytic infiltrate

Outcome: Fatality 8% (secondary to adrenal insufficiency)

LANGERHANS CELL HISTIOCYTOSIS (LCH)

CNS presentation: Typically presents with diabetes insipidus

- Temporal bone involvement common and may lead to a chronically draining ear

Radiology: Classically results in an enhancing lesion of the pituitary stalk and/or hypothalamic/chiasmal region

- Homogeneous on T1 and T2 weighted images
- May cause nonspecific brain parenchymal lesions, usually along perivascular spaces, but this is far less common

Pathology: Infiltrates composed of Langerhans cells (LCs), macrophages, lymphocytes, plasma cells, and mature eosinophils

- Birbeck granules on electron microscopy

Treatment: Radiation for isolated sellar region disease

- Chemotherapy and steroids for systemic disease (it often involves the bone, lung, and liver)

▓ Eosinophilic Granuloma
Solitary LCH lesion of skull or spine

▓ Hand-Schüller-Christian Disease
Multifocal LCH in bone and hypothalamus

■ Letterer-Siwe Disease
Multifocal disease involving skin, lymph nodes, viscera, and rarely the CNS

METASTASES

Epidemiology: Most common tumor to involve the brain

- Some studies quote 25% of all cancer patients at some point in the disease process will develop CNS metastases
- Secondary to hematogenous spread
- Most common tumors to metastasize to the brain are lung, breast, prostate, melanoma, renal, and colon cancers
- Metastases with a high propensity to hemorrhage include thyroid, choriocarcinoma, renal cell, lung, and melanoma

Radiology: Often multiple, commonly at gray-white junction

- May be ring enhancing or homogeneous
- May have cysts and hemorrhage
- Frequently associated with significant vasogenic edema

Treatment: Surgery, radiosurgery, and whole brain irradiation

- Solitary lesions that are surgically accessible are often resected followed by whole brain radiation (stereotactic radiosurgery is an alternative approach) while multiple lesions are often treated with whole brain irradiation (depending on the number of lesions, some institutions will treat with radiosurgery up front and save whole brain radiation for recurrence or progressive disease)
- Steroids for treatment of vasogenic edema

Outcome: Depends on tumor type, age, Karnofsky score, number of metastases, and whether primary disease is controlled

- Surgical resection improves outcome for solitary lesions

■ Dural and Leptomeningeal Metastases
Carcinomatous meningitis (leptomeningeal metastatic disease) is most common with lung and breast cancer

- Thickening and variable nodularity of leptomeninges, often best appreciated in IACs and over brainstem and cerebellar folia
- Hematogenous metastases to the dura may also occur and present as dural plaques that mimic meningioma

CYSTS

ARACHNOID CYST

Etiology: Nonneoplastic, developmental abnormality due to separation of the arachnoid membrane → wall thickens with collagen deposition

Pathophysiology: Active CSF secretion from cyst membrane, osmotic gradient, ball-valve mechanism

Location: Most commonly found in the middle fossa

Radiology: Follows CSF on all sequences, no enhancement

- Low signal on diffusion weighted imaging (distinct from epidermoid)

BOBBLE-HEAD DOLL SYNDROME

Pathophysiology: Dilated 3rd ventricle due to suprasellar arachnoid cyst distortion of the red nucleus and dentatorubrothalamic pathway, with compression on medial thalamus

Symptoms: Macrocephaly, ocular disturbance, psychomotor retardation, endocrine dysfunction

COLLOID CYST

Location: Usually in anterior/superior portion of 3rd ventricle between fornices at foramen of Monro

- Attached to the roof of the 3rd ventricle

Pathology: Outer fibrous layer, inner layer of simple cuboidal versus pseudostratified epithelium

- May derive from endodermal tissue of the paraphysis (vestigial remnant of 3rd ventricle structure)

Radiology: Dense on CT, bright on T1 due to high protein content

- Variably hypointense on T2
- Typically nonenhancing
- May be associated with obstructive hydrocephalus

Treatment: Surgery for size > 7 mm or symptomatic

Outcome: Has been associated with sudden death (acute obstructive hydrocephalus)

EPIDERMOID CYST

Epidemiology: Up to 2% of brain tumors

- Usually seen in adults

Pathophysiology: Ectopic ectodermal cells retained within the neural groove at 3–5 wks gestation

- Rupture may lead to aseptic meningitis (versus dermoid cyst which can lead to bacterial meningitis)

Location: Most commonly at cerebellopontine angle

- Also suprasellar/parasellar, middle fossa, prepontine cistern
- May be associated with dermal sinuses, usually along spine in kids

Radiology: Lobulated, slightly irregular margin

- Similar to CSF on CT and T1/T2 weighted images
- Very bright signal on diffusion-weighted images (epidermoid → hyper versus arachnoid cysts → hypo)
- Nonenhancing with contrast

Pathology: Fibrous capsule, "pearly tumor"

- Keratin and cholesterol crystals in center of lesion, squamous epithelium

DERMOID CYST

Epidemiology: 0.3% of brain tumors

- M > F
- More common in pediatric population
- Rupture may lead to acute clinical presentation with chemical meningitis (*Mollaret's meningitis*)
- May be associated with cutaneous tracts (skull base, occipital region, spine)
- May be associated with other congenital malformations (e.g., spinal dysraphism)
- Generally present at an earlier age than epidermoids

Location: Typically midline

- Lumbosacral spine > > parasellar > floor of anterior cranial fossa/nasal > posterior fossa

Radiology: Generally rounded and well circumscribed

- Typically bright on T1 weighted images due to fat content
- Suppresses on fat saturation images
- If ruptured, then fat globules may be seen distributed throughout the subarachnoid space

Pathology: Epithelial and dermoid elements: dermal appendages, hair follicles, macrophages, giant cells, sebaceous glands, sweat glands

- Inclusion of ectodermal elements in neural ectoderm during neurulation

Treatment: Surgical resection

CHOLESTEROL GRANULOMA/CYST

Symptoms: Headache, CNVI dysfunction

Location: Petrous apex

Pathophysiology: Chronic middle ear inflammation → obstruction of aerated petrous bone apex with accumulation of secretions and blood products

Radiology: Expansile lesion of petrous apex

- Bone thinning and lysis on CT

- Hyperintense on T1 and T2 weighted images
- No suppression on fat saturation images

Treatment: Surgical drainage if symptomatic or expanding

LEPTOMENINGEAL CYST

Uncommon complication of skull fracture in young child
- Simple skull fractures usually heal quickly in young children
- When skull fracture in infant or young child is complicated by dural tear, then the fracture may subsequently enlarge and present as a pulsatile mass
- Herniation of brain tissue into growing fracture may occur

Treatment: Excision and repair

PSEUDOMENINGOCELE

Collection of CSF caused by trauma, congenital, or postoperative
- Tear in the dura and leptomeninges such that CSF can leak out and accumulate in soft tissues and wall itself off, but it is not contained by dura as a true meningocele would be

Treatment: Observation, epidural blood patch, reoperation (repair of CSF leak), lumbar drain

OTHER

JUVENILE NASOPHARYNGEAL ANGIOFIBROMA

Usually arise along posterolateral nasal wall at the level of the sphenopalatine foramen
- Presentation typically nasal obstruction and variable epistaxis in teenage males
- Enlarged vascular channels in fibrovascular stroma
- Often extend to skull base
- Highly vascular, so do not biopsy

PARAGANGLIOMA (GLOMUS) TUMOR

In the head and neck and skull base, commonly occur at level of jugular bulb (glomus jugulare), cochlear promontory (glomus tympanicum), carotid sheath (glomus vagale), and carotid body (carotid body tumor)
- Heterogeneous, "salt-and-pepper" appearance on MRI due to prominent intratumoral flow voids
- Can secrete catecholamines/metanephrines
- Usually benign, but can be locally invasive
- Present variably with pulsatile tinnitus and/or hearing loss, lower cranial nerve deficits, neck mass

Treatment: Resection or irradiation (radiosurgery if small)

HAMARTOMA OF THE TUBER CINERUM[11]

Mass of ectopic cerebral gray matter between the infundibulum and mammillary bodies that is isointense to gray matter on CT and on MR sequences

- Benign
- Typically presents in children with either precocious puberty (hypothalamic inhibition disrupted) or gelastic (laughing) seizures

Management: Observation

NASAL GLIOMA[12]

Rare benign congenital mass of heterotopic glial tissue that is typically located in the midline at the level of the nasal bridge or nasal root

- M > F
- Arises from an abnormal closure of the fonticulus frontalis → extracranial ectopic rest of glial tissue
- No intracranial connection (though may be connected to dura in 15%)

Management: Observation, surgical resection if enlarges

CHAPTER 9 ■ STEREOTACTIC RADIOSURGERY

Gordon Sakamoto, MD

INTRODUCTION

Image-guided delivery of radiation to a defined target each individual beam carries a low dose of radiation, but the targeted area lies within the intersection of multiple beams and thus receives a much higher dose of radiation
- Primary or adjunct treatment

Benefits: Noninvasive, precise, accurate, good for deep lesions, no risks of anesthesia, outpatient, limited to no pain

Limitations: Size of lesion (> 3 cm), requires immobilization (stereotactic frame or mask)

INDICATIONS

Tumors (metastases [brain and spine], vestibular schwannoma, meningioma, pituitary adenomas, craniopharyngiomas, chordomas, and chondrosarcomas), vascular malformation (AVM >> arteriovenous fistulas), trigeminal neuralgia, tremor, epilepsy, cluster headaches, obsessive-compulsive disorder (OCD), and pain.

TYPES OF RADIOSURGERY

Depends on source of radiation:
1. Cobalt-60 based (Gamma Knife)
2. Linear accelerator (LINAC) based (Trilogy, CyberKnife)
3. Particle beam based (proton beam and heavy-ion beam)

COBALT-60 BASED (GAMMA KNIFE)

- Employs 201 cobalt-60 sources that are arranged in a semispherical array and a stereotactic frame that is affixed to the patient's skull.
- Uses isocentric planning to achieve conformality (a measure of how well the plan conforms to the shape of the target). Isocentric planning employs a method where the beams used to treat the lesion have a common focus point, or isocenter. By using isocenters of varying diameters, irregularly shaped lesions may be targeted with a high degree of conformality.

101

- Employs forward planning, in which a treatment plan is selected by an iterative trial-and-error approach.
- Requires a stereotactic frame and, therefore, can only treat intracranial pathology and cannot be fractionated.

LINEAR ACCELERATOR BASED

- Do not employ stereotactic frames.
- Can treat lesions outside of the head and neck.
- Can fractionate the total radiation dose over 2 to 5 days. Fractionation may protect the surrounding tissue by giving smaller doses of radiation during each session. The total dose is higher, but given in smaller amounts.

▓ Triology

- LINAC-based radiosurgical unit that uses a rotating gantry to deliver radiation. The gantry and the couch can move, but have limited degrees of motion.
- Frameless and can adjust for patient movement.
- Employs a multileaf collimator to shape the beams of radiation that it delivers. All other systems use collimators to produce round beams of radiation. The Trilogy uses shaped beams to produce a high degree of conformality.

▓ CyberKnife

- 6 MeV LINAC mounted on a robotic arm to deliver radiation. The robotic arm has 6° of freedom and moves around the patient.
- Uses wall-mounted X-rays to check the patient's position during treatment. Once a change in position has been detected, the robotic arm corrects the treatment plan for the change.
- Employs isocentric as well as nonisocentric planning to achieve conformality.
- Planning requires a specialized CT scan. Other images (MRI, CT Angio, etc.) may be fused to this CT to aid in target definition.
- Employs inverse planning in which the treating physician or surgeon specifies the target, dose, critical regions, and the relative importance of each, and the computer runs an optimization algorithm to find the best treatment plan.

PARTICLE BEAM BASED

Consists of proton-beam therapy and heavy-ion beam therapy.

▓ Proton-Beam Therapy

- Uses of protons accelerated with a particle accelerator and then aimed at the target.
- Protons are actually deposited into the target tissue and have no exit dose of radiation. Additionally, the maximum radiation dosage to the tissue occurs over the last few millimeters of the proton's range.
- This depth at which the proton deposits is dependent on the amount of energy imparted to the proton by the particle accelerator.
- Proton-beam therapy has been used for many different tumors, including chordomas, chondrosarcomas, and nasopharyngeal carcinomas.
- Proton-beam therapy is given over many sessions.

■ **Heavy-Ion Therapy**
Similar to proton-beam therapy, but uses larger ions such as helium and carbon.

SIDE EFFECTS

- Nausea, vomiting (area postrema)
- Hair loss
- Cerebral edema
- Radiation injury to adjacent structures, demyelination
- Radiation necrosis (affects mainly white matter; necrosis is due to small artery injury and thrombotic occlusion)
- Secondary tumors (astrocytoma, meningioma, sarcoma)
- Telangiectasia/cavernous malformation
- Mineralizing microangiopathy, vasculopathy/Moyamoya

CHAPTER 10 ■ NEUROENDOCRINOLOGY[1-5]

Jason Davies, MD

ADDISON'S DISEASE[6,7]

- Chronic adrenal insufficiency, hypocortisolism (glucocorticoids and mineralocorticoids)

Symptoms/Signs: Fatigue, muscle weakness, arthralgia, weight loss, emesis, diarrhea, headache, diaphoresis, mood changes, salt craving, skin hyperpigmentation, orthostatic hypotension, goiter, vitiligo

- Can be life threatening if in Addisonian crisis (refractory hemodynamic instability, pain, psychosis, seizures)

Diagnostics: Hypoglycemia, hyponatremia, hyperkalemia, hypoglycemia, eosinophilia, lymphocytosis, metabolic acidosis (low aldosterone stimulation of the renal distal tubule leads to urine sodium wasting and H+ retention)

- ACTH (cortrosyn) stimulation test, cortisol level, fasting blood sugar
Treatment: Cortisol replacement therapy (hydrocortisone/prednisone)
- Some may need fludrocortisone to replace aldosterone
- May require increased doses during times of stress, injury, or infection

CUSHING'S SYNDROME

- Prolonged exposure to high blood levels of cortisol
- Also known as hyperadrenocorticism or hypercorticism

Etiologies: Iatrogenic, benign or malignant adrenal neoplasm, ectopic ACTH-secreting neoplasm (esp. lungs, thyroid, thymus, pancreas), pituitary adenoma (Cushing's disease), depression, and chronic alcoholism (pseudo-Cushing's syndrome)

Symptoms/Signs: Rapid weight gain; increased appetite; hypertension; rounded "moon" facies; facial flushing; increased fat deposits in abdomen, neck (buffalo hump), and back; stretch marks (abdominal striae); poor wound healing; skin thinning; fatigue; muscle and bone weakness; menstrual abnormalities; depression, severe mood swings

Diagnostics: 24-hour urine free-cortisol with creatinine and creatinine clearance, serum cortisol, ACTH levels, low-dose decadron suppression test, late night salivary or serum cortisol level, CRH stimulation tests

- If tests confirm hypercortisolemia and indicate pituitary source of excess ACTH, may perform CT/MRI (but note that 10% of population has incidental pituitary abnormality)
- If tests inconclusive, inferior petrosal sinus sampling (IPPS) study may be performed to confirm central source and suggest affected side of gland

Treatment: See Table 10-1.

Table 10-1 Treatment of Cushing Syndrome

Etiology	Treatment
Iatrogenic	Taper offending medication
Adrenal adenoma	Surgical resection followed by steroid replacement
	Pharmacotherapy to inhibit cortisol synthesis (e.g., ketoconazole, metyrapone)
Pituitary adenoma	Transsphenoidal resection followed by steroid replacement

SYNDROME OF INAPPROPRIATE ANTI-DIURETIC HORMONE SECRETION (SIADH)[8]

- Release of ADH not inhibited by decreased plasma osmolality
- Results in dilutional hyponatremia
- Normo- or HYPERvolemia

Etiologies: Meningitis, SAH, lung cancer, brain abscess, pneumonia, lung abscess, drugs (chlorpropamide, clofibrate, phenothiazine, cyclosphosphamide, carbamazepine, SSRIs, MDMA)

Symptoms/Signs: Hyponatremia, ECF volume expansion without edema or hypertension, natriuresis, headache, nausea, emesis

- Severe hyponatremia ($P_{Na} < 120$ mOsm) leads to cerebral edema: irritability, confusion, convulsions, coma
- Concentrated (high urine specific gravity), low urine output

Diagnostics: $P_{Na} < 130$ mEq/L, $P_{Osm} < 270$ mOsm, $U_{Osm} > 300$ mOsm, $U_{Na} > 20$ mEq/L, HYPERvolemia (elevated CVP), suppression of renin-angiotensin system, low BUN, low creatinine, low uric acid, low albumin

- Water restriction challenge: Increase in P_{Na} implies SIADH

Treatment: Treat underlying cause

- Fluid restriction (0.8–1 L/day)
- Hypertonic saline if severely symptomatic (3% gtt)
- Drugs: Demeclocycline (most potent ADH inhibitor), conivaptan (V_{1a} and V_2 antagonist), tolvaptan (V_2 antagonist), furosemide, salt tabs

- NOTE: Rapid rise in P_{Na} level may cause central pontine myelinolysis, therefore, goal change < 10 mEq/L/day

CEREBRAL SALT WASTING SYNDROME[9]

- Excessive natriuresis with subsequent hyponatremic dehydration
- Centrally mediated process in patients with intracranial disease
- Relative or overt HYPOvolemia

Etiologies: Head injury, intracranial neoplasm, intracranial surgery, intracranial hemorrhage, CVA, tuberculous meningitis, craniosynostosis repair

Symptoms/Signs: Dehydration, hypovolemia, thirst, abrupt weight loss, decreasing urinary frequency, negative fluid balance

- Cerebral edema: Lethargy, agitation, headache, altered mental status, seizures, coma

Diagnostics: Hyponatremia, large volume UOP, $U_{Na} > 100$ mEq/L, hypovolemic (e.g., low CVP)

Treatment: Correct intravascular volume depletion and hyponatremia

- Hypertonic saline for replacement of ongoing urinary sodium loss
- Fludrocortisone
- Enteral salt supplementation once stablilized

CENTRAL DIABETES INSIPIDUS

Etiologies: Neurogenic— lack of vasopressin production

- Dipsogenic— defect or damage to thirst mechanism in hypothalamus
- Commonly associated with germinomas, Langerhans cell histiocytosis, lymphocytic hypophysitis, craniopharyngiomas, pituitary adenomas

Symptoms/Signs: Excessive thirst

- Large volume, highly diluted urine despite high serum osmolarity
- No impact of fluid restriction
- Blurred vision
- Dehydration, HYPOvolemia

Diagnostics: Normal serum glucose, bicarbonate, calcium

- Hypernatremia, low urine specific gravity, low urine osmolarity, urine electrolytes low
- Fluid deprivation test: Continues to urinate large volumes of dilute urine

Treatment: Desmopressin (DDAVP), adequate hydration

PITUITARY DYSFUNCTION AND NEOPLASMS[10,11]

CLASSIFICATION

■ Adenomas
Benign tumors in or on pituitary
- Named based on size and ability to secrete hormones

Functioning Tumors
Produce excessive amounts of pituitary hormone (see Table 10-2)
- Symptoms depend on type of hormone produced
- Usually diagnosed when small due to high hormone levels

Nonfunctioning Tumors
Do not produce hormones
- Symptoms produced by mass effect (e.g., on optic chiasm)
- Symptoms include visual changes (field loss or diplopia), headache, impaired sexual function, lack of energy

Microadenoma
≤ 1 cm diameter
- Most commonly microprolactinomas

Macroadenoma
> 1 cm diameter
- Headache and visual field cuts most frequent symptoms

Table 10-2 Pituitary Hormones

	Hormone	Target Organ(s)	Physiologic Effect
Anterior pituitary: Controlled by hypothalamus by way of secretions into hypothalamic-hypophyseal portal system	Growth hormone (GH)	Liver, adipose tissue	Promotes growth; control of protein, lipid, carbohydrate metabolism
	Thyroid-stimulating hormone (TSH)	Thyroid	Stimulates secretion of thyroid hormones
	Adenocorticotropic hormone (ACTH)	Adrenal cortex	Stimulates secretion of glucocorticoids
	Prolactin (PL)	Mammary gland	Milk production
	Luteinizing hormone (LH)	Ovary/testis	Control of reproductive function
	Follicle-stimulating hormone (FSH)	Ovary/testis	Control of reproductive function
Posterior pituitary: aka neurohypophysis, a collection of axonal projections from the hypothalamus.	Antidiuretic hormone (ADH)	Kidney	Conservation of body water
	Oxytocin	Uterus, breast	Parturition, lactation

▦ Other Intrasellar Masses

Nonpituitary Adenoma Intra-/Suprasellar Masses

Abscess, arachnoid cysts, chordoma, coccidioidomycosis, craniopharyngioma (arises from nests of epithelium from Rathke's pouch filled with cholesterol fluid, calcifications) cysticercosis, dermoid cysts, epidermoid cysts, empty sella syndrome, germ cell tumors, granular cell tumors, lymphocytic hypophysitis, lymphoma, meningiomas, meningoencephaloceles, mucoceles, pituitary astrocytomas, plasmacytoma, Rathke's cleft cyst, rhabdomyosarcomas, sarcoidosis

▦ Apoplexy

Pituitary Apoplexy

Sudden onset of gland failure or neurological deficits

- Due to hemorrhage or infarction
- Most commonly occurs in macroadenomas
- Common symptoms: Headache, nausea, emesis, visual changes, altered mental status, meningismus

PROLACTINOMA[12]

Benign prolactin-producing neoplasm

- May be micro- or macroprolactinomas

▦ Microprolactinomas

Elevate serum prolactin to < 150 mg/ml

- Most common in premenopausal women

▦ Macroadenomas

1–2 cm can elevate serum prolactin to 200–1000 ng/ml

- > 2 cm can elevate serum prolactin to > 1000 ng/ml

Symptoms/Signs: Amenorrhea, galactorrhea, diminished libido, vaginal dryness, infertility, headaches, visual changes, osteoporosis, mood changes, depression

Diagnostics: Hyperprolactinema (> 150 ng/ml)

- Complete pituitary hormone evaluation
- DDx of elevated prolactin: Pregnancy or postpartum, stress, hypothyroidism, renal failure, liver failure, medications, "stalk effect" (elevation of serum prolactin levels by nonhormone-producing tumors due to pressure on pituitary stalk that interferes with transport of inhibitory dopamine to pituitary from hypothalamus)
- "Hook effect": Erroneously low serum prolactin levels in patients with very large prolactinoms; serum dilution reveals much higher prolactin levels

Treatment: Most respond to medical treatment

- Usually lifelong bromocriptine or cabergoline for control
- If fails to respond or unable to tolerate medication, proceed to surgery

- Surgery is primary treatment for macroademonas with prolactin < 200 ng/ml

ACROMEGALY AND GIGANTISM[1]

Benign tumor producing excess GH

▚ Acromegaly

Tumor develops after normal growth has ended

- Enlargement of hands, feet, head, jaw, internal organs

▚ Gigantism

Tumor develops before growth plates close

- Enlargement of hands, feet, head, jaw, internal organs, coarse facial features, enlarged lips, nose, tongue, snoring, excessive diaphoresis, oily skin, fatigue, weakness, arthritis, arthralgias, hypertension, low libido, impotence, amenorrhea, depression, visual changes, diabetes, arteriosclerosis, carpal tunnel syndrome, polyps

Treatment: Primary treatment is transsphenoidal resection

- Radiosurgery
- Medical therapy (e.g., somatostatin analogs, dopamine agonists, GH receptor antagonists)
- Radiation therapy

THYROID-STIMULATING HORMONE (TSH) SECRETING TUMOR

Rare

- May be micro- or macroadenomas
- Rare cause of hyperthyroidism
- More difficult to resect

CHAPTER 11 ■ NEURORADIOLOGY

Anthony Wang, MD
Melanie G. Hayden Gephart, MD, MAS

Table 11-1 Differential Diagnosis by Location and Imaging Characteristics of Intracranial Neoplasms[1,2]

Location	Tumor	T1	T1c	T2	Comments
Lobar					
	Metastasis	Hypo/Iso	++	Iso/Hyper	Often cystic or hemorrhagic; typically extensive edema
	GBM	Hypo/Iso	++	Iso/Hyper	Often involve corpus callosum; ring >> solid enhancement; often cystic or hemorrhagic; + edema
	Oligodendroglioma	Hypo/Iso	50/50	Hyper	Frontal > other; involves cortex; calcifications common
	Grade II/III Astrocytoma	Hypo	Varies	Hyper	More enhancement as grade increases; edema usually w/ grade II, variable w/ grade III
	Ganglioglioma	Hypo/Iso	Varies	Hyper	Often cysts, calcification; cortical location; seizures
	DNET	Hypo	+/-	Hyper	Often multiple cysts, nodular enhancement; cortical; seizures
	PNET	Hypo/Iso	+	Iso; cysts hyper	Heterogeneous; variable edema; usually children
	Atypical teratoid–rhabdoid tumor	Iso	+	Iso/hyper	Children < 3 yrs; heterogeneity (cysts, hemorrhage, necrosis); large
Non-neoplastic "mimics"	Tumefactive demyelination	Hypo/Iso	+	Hyper/Iso	Less mass effect for size than neoplasm; "open ring" of incomplete enhancement
	Infection (abscess)	Hypo/Iso	++	Hyper	Appearance varies by etiology; pyogenic = ring-enhancing with large edema, DWI bright

Pineal Region[3]					
Pineal gland	Germinoma	Iso	++	Iso	Usually homogeneous
	Teratoma	Varies	50/50	Varies	Heterogeneous; often cysts, calcification, fat
	Embryonal cell carcinoma	Hypo/Iso	+	Hyper/Iso	Heterogeneous; adolescents
	Pineocytoma	Hypo/Iso	+	Iso/Hyper	Round, often calcified, heterogeneous; brain edema uncommon
	Pineoblastoma (PNET)	Hypo/Iso	+	Iso	Usually young children; associated with retinoblastoma; calcification uncommon, edema+
	Pineal cyst	Hypo	-	Hyper	Usually incidental; residual gland enhances around margin
	Astrocytoma (supporting cells)	Hypo/Iso	Varies w/ grade	Hyper	
Brainstem	Tectal glioma	Hypo/Iso	Uncommon	Hyper	Often benign pathologically, but unresectable; locally invasive
Quadrigeminal cistern	Arachnoid cyst	Iso to CSF	-	Iso to CSF	Sharply demarcated; like CSF on DWI (low signal intensity)
	Epidermoid cyst	Hypo	-	Hyper	Irregular margin; very bright on DWI
	Dermoid cyst	Hyper	-	Varies	Fat components suppress w/ fat saturation; may rupture into subarachnoid space
Intraventricular					
Frontal horns	Giant cell astrocytoma	Hypo/Iso	++	Iso/Hyper	Arise from foramen of Monro; associated w/ tuberous sclerosis

(Continued)

Table 11-1 Differential Diagnosis by Location and Imaging Characteristics of Intracranial Neoplasms [1,2] (continued)

Location	Tumor	T1	T1c	T2	Comments
Intraventricular					
Body of lateral ventricles	Central neurocytoma	Iso	+	Hyper	"Feathery" enhancement; attached to septum pellucidum
	Subependymoma	Hypo/Iso	Varies	Hyper	Older patients; lobulated lesion
	Oligodendroglioma	Hypo/Iso	50/50	Hyper	Rare in this location; many reclassified as central neurocytoma
Atria of lateral ventricles	Choroid plexus papilloma	Hypo/Iso	++	Hyper/Iso	Most common location in children; highly vascular
	Metastasis	Iso	++	Iso/Hyper	Usually to choroid plexus
	Meningioma	Iso	++	Iso	More common in older woman, usually on L
	Choroid plexus cyst	Iso to CSF	-	Iso to CSF	Commonly bilateral; incidental finding; low on DWI (iso to CSF)
	Choroid plexus xanthogranuloma	Hypo/Iso	-	Varies	Often bilateral; incidental finding in older patients; often bright on DWI
Foramen of Monro and 3rd ventricle	Colloid cyst	Hyper	-	Iso/Hyper	Anterosuperior 3rd ventricle; round; usually dense on noncontrast CT
	Metastasis	Iso	++	Iso	Met to choroid plexus
	Choroid plexus papilloma	Hypo/Iso	++	Iso/Hyper	Young children; very rare location; highly vascular
	Subependymal giant cell astrocytoma	Hypo/Iso	++	Hyper/Iso	Typically associated w/ tuberous sclerosis; heterogeneous
	Germinoma	Iso	++	Iso/Hyper	More common in young patients

Location	Lesion	T1	T2	Enhancement	Comments
	Meningioma	Hypo/Iso	Iso	++	Arises from tentorium or lower falx
	Ependymoma	Hypo/Iso	Hyper/Iso	+	Rare location; lobulated intraventricular mass
Aqueduct	Tectal glioma	Hypo/Iso	Hyper	50/50	Often indolent; often assoc w/ NF1
	Subependymoma	Hypo/Iso	Hyper	Varies	4th ventricular location most common
	Hemangio-blastoma	Iso	Hyper	++	Rare location, flow voids if lesion large
4th ventricle	See Cerebellopontine Angle (CPA)				
All	High-grade astrocytoma	Hypo/Iso	Iso/Hyper	Incr w/ grade	Usually due to gross extension into ventricles and/or subependymal spread
Cerebellopontine Angle (CPA)					
Cistern	8th nerve schwannoma	Hypo/Iso	Hyper (Hypo to CSF)	++	Most common mass lesion of CPA; typically bilateral in NF-2
	Meningioma	Hypo/Iso	Iso	++	Broad dural base; may be calcified
	Epidermoid cyst	Hypo	Hyper	-	Bright on DWI; often irregular margin
	Arachnoid cyst	Hypo	Hyper	-	Follows CSF on DWI; smooth margin
Internal auditory canal	8th nerve schwannoma (acoustic neuroma)	Iso	Hyper (hypo to CSF)	++	Classic: "ice cream cone" shape of IAC and CPA components
Cerebellopontine Angle (CPA)					
4th ventricle/lateral recess	Ependymoma	Hypo/Iso	Hyper/Iso	+	Typically arises from floor, lobulated; extension through foramina of Luschka and Magendie common
	Choroid plexus papilloma	Hypo/Iso	Hyper/Iso	++	Most common location in adults; multilobulated lesion

(Continued)

Table 11-1 Differential Diagnosis by Location and Imaging Characteristics of Intracranial Neoplasms:[1,2] (continued)

Location	Tumor	T1	T1c	T2	Comments
	Medulloblastoma	Iso	+	Iso	Classically arises from roof; CSF spread common
	Low-grade astrocytoma	Hypo/Iso	Variable	Iso/Hyper	Includes dorsally exophytic brainstem glioma and ventrally exophytic cerebellar pilocytic astrocytoma
	Metastasis	Hypo/Iso	++	Iso/Hyper	Typically metastasis to choroid plexus; rarely leptomeningeal[4]
Brainstem and cerebellum	Astrocytoma, grades 2 to 4	Hypo/Iso	50/50	Iso/Hyper	Enhancement, heterogeneity increase w/ grade
	Pilocytic astrocytoma	Hypo/Iso	++	Hyper	Typically cystic w/ enhancing mural nodule; children
	Medulloblastoma	Hypo/Iso	+	Iso	Cerebellar hemisphere location seen in teens/adults
	Hemangioblastoma	Iso	++	Hyper	Larger lesions cystic w/ enhancing mural nodule; associated with VHL
	Atypical teratoid-rhabdoid tumor	Iso	+	Varies	Usually off midline: cysts, hemorrhage frequent; may mimic medulloblastoma
	Dysplastic gangliocytoma (Lhermitte–Duclos dz)	Hypo/Iso	Rare	Hyper	Striated appearance; associated with Cowden syndrome
Sellar Region					
Sellar	Pituitary microadenoma	Iso	+	Iso/Hyper	Typically enhances less than surrounding gland on dynamic imaging; < 10 mm
	Pituitary macroadenoma	Iso	++	Iso/Hyper	Can be cystic or hemorrhagic; ≥ 10 mm; classically enlarges sella, extends into suprasellar cistern

Suprasellar	Cyst (Rathke's cleft or pars intermedia)	Varies/Hypo	-	Varies/Hyper	Appearance varies w/ protein content of cyst; often extends to suprasellar cistern
	Craniopharyngioma	Varies	+	Hyper	Usually mixed cystic and solid; calcification on CT; cysts often bright on T1WI
	Meningioma	Iso	++	Iso	Separate from pituitary gland; often tuberculum
	Hypothalamic/Chiasmal glioma	Iso	Varies	Hyper/Iso	Pilocytic astrocytoma
(Nonneoplastic)	Epidermoid cyst	Hypo	-	Hyper	Very bright on DWI; lobulated, slightly irregular
	Dermoid cyst	Hyper	-	Varies	May rupture into subarachnoid space; fat content suppresses w/ fat sat
	Lipoma	Hyper	-	Iso to fat	Follow fat on all sequences; often partly calcified
	Arachnoid cyst	Iso to CSF	-	Iso to CSF	Sharply demarcated; like CSF on DWI
	Aneurysm	Varies	Varies	Varies	Highly variable signal: heterogeneous, lamellated, flow void, phase artifact
Infundibulum	Germinoma	Iso	+	Iso	Typically present with diabetes insipidus
	Lymphoma/Leukemia	Iso	+	Iso	Often other sites of CNS involvement
Sellar Region	Sarcoid	Iso	+	Iso	Associated w/ hilar adenopathy, elevated ACE level
	Histiocytosis	Iso	+	Iso	Associated w/ lytic bone lesions
	Metastasis	Iso	+	Iso/Hyper	Often other lesions
	Pituicytoma/Choristoma	Hypo/Iso	Varies	Hypo/Iso	Posterior pituitary, infudibular; rare

(Continued)

Table 11-1 Differential Diagnosis by Location and Imaging Characteristics of Intracranial Neoplasms[1,2] (continued)

Location	Tumor	T1	T1c	T2	Comments
Hypothalamic/Chiasmal	Astrocytoma[5]	Hypo/Iso	Varies	Hyper	Often pilocytic and associated with NF1; variable cysts, hemorrhage uncommon
	Germinoma	Hypo/Iso	++	Hyper/Iso	
	Metastasis	Hypo/Iso	++	Hyper/Iso	
(Nonneoplastic)	Hamartoma	Iso	-	Iso	Tuber cinereum, sessile or pedunculated; follows gray matter
Cavernous sinus	Meningioma	Iso	++	Iso	Often a dural tail extending along skull base; hyperostosis
	Schwannoma	Iso	+	Hyper	Rounded, well circumscribed; cysts common
	Metastasis	Iso	+	Iso/Hyper	More infiltrative than meningioma
	Pituitary adenoma	Iso	+	Iso	Usually extension of a sellar lesion
	Lymphoma	Iso	++	Iso	Can be identical to metastasis, sarcoid, LCH; often bilateral
Nonneoplastic	Infection	Iso		Iso/Hyper	Low or iso on T2 if fungal
	Tolosa Hunt (orbital inflammatory) syndrome	Iso	+	Iso	Commonly presents with retroorbital pain; cavernous ICA may be narrowed
	Cavernous sinus thrombosis	Iso	-	Iso/Hyper	Filling defect in sinus; bland vs. septic (often assoc w/ infection)
Skull Base					
Anterior (frontal sinuses, cribriform plate, ethmoid roof), central (sphenoid bone, basiocciput), and posterolateral (temporal bone, jugular foramen)					
Anterior skull base	Squamous cell carcinoma	Iso	+	Iso	Most arise from maxillary sinus; bone destruction common

	Rhabdomyosarcoma	Hypo/Iso	++	Iso	Peak incidence 2–5 years of age[6]
	Esthesioneuroblastoma	Iso	+	Iso	Typically arise in olfactory recess; may see peripheral cysts w/ intracranial extension
	Adenoid cystic carcinoma	Iso	+	Iso/Hyper	Infiltrative; perineural spread of disease
	Inverted papilloma[6,7]	Hypo/Iso	+	Iso/Hyper	Lateral nasal wall or sinus origin; cerebriform pattern
	Meningioma	Iso	++	Iso	Along planum sphenoidale or olfactory groove
(Nonneoplastic)	Metastasis	Hypo/Iso	++	Iso/Hyper	May arise from bone or dura
	Mucocele	Hyper	- (unless infected)	Varies	Well-defined expansile mass; signal intensity varies w/ protein content, viscosity[6]
	Nasoethmoidal cephalocele	Hypo/Iso	-	Iso/Hyper	CSF +/- brain; signal characteristics depend on contents
Central skull base	Chordoma	Hypo	+	Hyper	Typically midline, arises from clivus
Skull Base					
	Chondrosarcoma	Hypo	++	Hyper	Typically off-midline, petro-clival fissure
	Metastasis	Iso	++	Iso	Bone destruction, irregular margin
	Myeloma	Hypo	+	Hyper	
(Superior extension to central skull base)	Nasopharyngeal carcinoma	Iso	+	Iso	Often extends to clivus; nodal metastases
	Juvenile nasopharyngeal angiofibroma	Iso	++	Iso/Hyper	Teenage males; visible flow voids

(Continued)

Table 11-1 Differential Diagnosis by Location and Imaging Characteristics of Intracranial Neoplasms [1,2] (continued)

Location	Tumor	T1	T1c	T2	Comments
(Inferior extension to central skull base)	Pituitary adenoma	Iso	++	Iso	May extend to clivus, sphenoid sinus
	Meningioma	Iso	++	Iso	Dural base; hyperostosis; common along sphenoid wing
(Nonneoplastic)	Sinusitis	Varies	+	Varies	If fungal, often dark on T2; heterogeneous signal intensity
Posterolateral skull base	Metastasis	Hypo/Iso	++	Iso/Hyper	Irregular, bone destruction, often multiple
	Meningioma	Hypo/Iso	++	Iso	Dural based, may be calcified
(Nonneoplastic)	Osteomyelitis	Hypo/Iso	++	Iso/Hyper	Marrow space infection
Petrous apex	Cholesterol granuloma	Hyper	-	Hyper	Expansile lesion of petrous apex
	Cholesteatoma	Hypo/Iso	-	Hyper	High signal on DWI
	Chondrosarcoma[a]	Hypo/Iso	++	Hyper	Extend laterally from petroclival fissure
Posterior petrous face	Endolymphatic sac tumor[a]	Varies	+	Varies	Hypervascular, heterogeneous, associated w/ VHL
Jugular foramen	Schwannoma	Iso	++	Hyper	Smooth remodeling of bone
	Meningioma	Hypo/Iso	++	Iso	Dural based, often calcified
	Paraganglioma	Iso	++	Iso/Hyper	Flow voids, irregular margin
	Metastasis	Hypo/Iso	++	Iso/Hyper	Bone destruction, pain

Dural/Leptomeningeal					
	Meningioma	Hypo/Iso	++	Iso	Hyperostosis, dural based, dural tail
	Metastasis	Hypo/Iso	++	Hyper/Iso	May be associated with bone erosion
	Hemangiopericytoma	Iso	++	Iso	Mimics meningioma, more lobulated, less broad dural base
(Nonneoplastic)	Infection	Iso	+	Iso	Appearance varies by etiology
	Sarcoidosis	Iso	++	Iso	Nodular infiltration of dura, leptomeninges; may involve parenchyma, usually extending along perivascular spaces
	Tuberculosis	Iso	++	Hypo	Variable enhancement
	Histiocytosis	Iso	++	Hyper	Can look similar to sarcoid; often involves temporal bone, causes bone erosion
	Lymphoma/Leukemia	Iso	++	Iso	Mimics other nonspecific infiltrative lesions (e.g., metastases, sarcoid)

NOTE: Hypo/Iso/Hyperintensity are relative to brain parenchyma, typically gray matter

GBM = glioblastoma multiforme, VHL = Von Hippel–Lindau, mets = metastases, LCH = Langerhans cell histiocytosis, ICA = internal carotid artery

Sources: Osborn[1], Osborn et al.[2]

(See Table 11-1 for further clinical details on the following neoplasms)

ASSORTED ADDITIONAL DIFFERENTIAL DIAGNOSES[9–11]

EXTRAAXIAL

▓ Skull Tumor
Dermoid, epidermoid, fibrous displasia, metastatic lesion, aneurysmal bone cyst, osteoma, osteoblastoma, osteoid osteoma, chordoma, fibrosarcoma, giant cell tumor
- "Pseudosubarachnoid hemorrhage," as is seen with severe increased ICP and low density brain, making meninges seem dense

▓ Wormian Bone
Multiple areas of ossification skull cranial sutures (lambdoidal, posterior sagittal, tempero-squamous)
- Normal up to 6 months of age
- Mnemonic: *PORKCCHOPS* = **P**ycnodysostosis, **O**steogenesis imperfecta, **R**ickets, **K**inky hair syndrome of Menke, **C**retinism, **C**liedocranial dysplasia, **H**ypophospatasia, **O**topalatodigital syndrome, **P**rimary acroosteolysis, pachydermoperiostosis, **S**yndromes, and chromosome disorder (e.g., Trisomy 21)

▓ Dural-Based Lesions
Meningioma, metastases, hemangiopericytoma, sarcoidosis, LCH, TB

▓ Increased Density in Subarachnoid Space on Noncontrast CT
Blood, pus, tumor

INTRAPARENCHYMAL

▓ Causes of Restricted Diffusion (DWI)[12]
- Arterial infarction: Due to cytotoxic edema. With true reduced diffusion, areas that are bright on DWI should be dark on the corresponding apparent diffusion coefficient (ADC) map. With vasogenic edema, there can be high signal on DWI due to "T2 shine-through" and ADC is not low.
- Venous infarction: Variable regions of reduced diffusion
- Abscess: Pyogenic abscess typically has central reduced diffusion
- Viral encephalitis: Notably HSV 1; reduced diffusion in affected cortex

Table 11-2 Hemorrhage Appearance on MRI

Stage	Time from Stroke	T1	T2
Hyperacute	0–6 hours	Isointense	Hyperintense
Acute	7–72 hours	Isointense	Hypointense
Early subacute	4–7 days	Hyperintense	Hypointense
Late subacute	1–4 weeks	Hyperintense	Hyperintense
Early chronic	weeks to months	Hyperintense	Hyperintense
Late chronic	months to years	Hypointense	Hypointense

- Prion disease (Creutzfeldt-Jakob disease): Variable reduced diffusion in cortical ribbon ("cortical ribboning") and in deep gray nuclei
- Acute demyelination (e.g., multiple sclerosis plaque – also bright on T2/Flair)
- Mitochondrial disease: Areas of acute injury show reduced diffusion
- Toxic/metabolic insult (e.g., methotrexate toxicity)
- Certain tumors: Typically those with high nuclear-to-cytoplasmic ratio such as lymphoma and other small round blue cell tumors
- Epidermoid cyst: Helpful in distinguishing from arachnoid cyst
- Hematoma (subacute hemorrhage)

Cerebral Calcifications
Idiopathic (basal ganglia, pineal gland), neoplastic (tumor, tuberous sclerosis), metabolic (hypo-/hyperparathyroid hormone), vascular (Sturge-Weber syndrome, postanoxic, posthemorrhage), inflammatory, developmental (Trisomy 13, Cockayne's disease), infectious (AIDS in kids; TORCH infection, CMV > rubella, toxoplasmosis, herpes simplex)

Ring-Enhancing Lesions
MAGIC DR → Metastatic, Abscess, Glioblastoma, Infarct, Contusion, Demyelination, Radionecrosis
- Also includes other infection (toxopasmosis, fungal infection, tuberculoma, parasitic), subacute infarct

Cystic Lesions
Neoplastic → pilocytic astrocytoma, desmoplastic infantile ganglioglioma, ependymoma (in spine, not so much in brain), hemangioblastoma, pleomorphic xanthoastrocytoma, craniopharyngioma, meningioma (rare), schwannoma (if large)
- Nonneoplastic → developmental cysts (epidermoid, arachnoid, choroid, colloid, Rathke, endodermal, ependymal)

Bilateral Thalamic Signal Abnormality
Vascular (arterial: artery of Percheron infarction, top of the basilar syndrome, vasculitis; venous: internal cerebral vein/vein of Galen/straight sinus occlusion or hypertension due to AVF); infectious (viral encephalitis, PML); demyelinating (ADEM, osmotic); metabolic (Wernicke encephalopathy, cytochrome C oxidase deficiency); neoplastic (astrocytoma, lymphoma)

Corpus Callosum
- Lesions that extend across the corpus callosum: GBM, lymphoma, demyelination (PML, Marchiafava-Bignami)
- Abnormal corpus callosum signal that resolves: Seizures, trauma, antiepileptic drugs, PRES, demyelination

---

MR SPECTROSCOPY[13]

Plots the relative concentration of a given metabolite versus the effect that the metabolite has on the rotational frequency of protons within the sample (measured in parts per million [ppm])

- Metabolite peaks have characteristic ppm locations on the x-axis, and the amplitudes of their respective peaks (y-axis) have characteristic relationships in normal and abnormal brain. (See Table 11-3)
- See also Table 11-4 for clinical applications.

Table 11-3 Most Important MR Spectroscopy Peaks

Marker	Location (ppm)	Significance
Lipid/Lactate	1.3	Inflammation, necrosis, anaerobic glycolysis
N-acetylaspartate (NAA)	2.0	Neuronal viability
Creatine	3.0	Energy metabolism; useful reference peak as generally stable
Glutamine/Glutamate (glx) (GABA)	2.2	Neuronal damage (astrocytes), neurotransmitters
Choline	3.2	Membrane turnover (phospholipid synthesis)

Table 11-4 Clinical Application of MR Spectroscopy

Category	Clinical Condition	Metabolite
Neoplasm	High-grade glial neoplasm	Increased: Choline, lactate, lipids; decreased: NAA
	Meningioma	Increased: Alanine, glutamates; decreased: creatine
	Metastases	Increased: Choline, lactate, lipids; decreased: NAA
	Lymphoma	Increased: Choline; decreased: NAA
Infection	Abscess	Increased: Lactate, succinate, alanine, acetate, lipids; low NAA
Metabolic	Ethanol use	Triplet
	Diabetic ketoacidosis	Glucose, acetone
	Maple syrup urine disease	Branched chain amino acids
	Galactosemia	Galactitol
	Phenylketonuria (PKU)	Phenylalanine
	Lipid storage disease	Lipids
	Canavan disease	NAA
	Leigh disease, MELAS	Lactate
	Peroxisomal disorder	Scyllo-inositol
Other	Radiation necrosis	Increased: Lipids, lactate, choline
	Alzheimer disease	Increased: Myoinositol; decreased: NAA
	Down syndrome	Increased: Myoinositol; decreased: NAA

NOTE: Can also see mannitol (after treatment for elevated ICP) at 3.88 ppm[14]

CHAPTER 12 ■ SPINE[1-5]

Melanie G. Hayden Gephart, MD, MAS
Scott Berta, MD

PHYSICAL EXAM[6]

Table 12-1 Physical Exam: Spine

Test	Description	Positive Findings
Adson's test[7]	Patient seated, arm dependent, neck toward side being tested and extended, deep breath. ↓ pulse is positive	↓ pulse = thoracic outlet syndrome
Babinski	Stroking the bottom of the foot causes reflex toe extension	Upper motor neuron lesion (normal in newborns)
Bowstring	Hip flexed to 90°, knee flexed to reduce radicular symptoms, pressure placed on tibial nerve in popliteal area	Reproduces radicular pain
Crossed straight leg raise	Passive lifting of contralateral straight leg, flex hip with straight knee	Suggests a herniated disc
Clonus	Forced dorsiflexion of the foot	Reflex rhythmic plantar flexion response > 4 beats
Femoral nerve traction test	Place the patient laterally on the unaffected side, examiner passively extends the hip and flexes the knee of the affected side	Reproduces radicular pain
Hoffman's	Flicking distal interphalangeal joint (DIPJ) of middle finger causes involuntary flexion of DIPJ of index and IPJ of thumb	Myelopathic sign
Lhermitte's	Forward flexion of neck causes lancinating pain down spinal cord	Stenotic sign
Straight leg raise	Passive lifting of straight leg, flex hip with straight knee, ± dorsiflexion of foot (Lesegue maneuver)	Reproduces radicular symptoms; dorsiflexion should reproduce symptoms at less hip flexion
Waddell's signs[8]	1. Pain (out of proportion) to superficial touch [superficial tenderness] 2. Pain with axial rotation of the pelvis and with axial loading on the top of the skull [simulation] 3. Sitting straight leg raise < lying SLR [distraction] 4. Nonanatomic weakness or sensory changes 5. Overreaction	May indicate heavy psychosocial overlay (three or more of five signs present)

125

Table 12-2 Simplified Exam and Corresponding Spinal Cord Level

Spinal Cord Level	Motor Exam (Muscle)	Motor Nerve	Reflex	Sensory Area	Sensory Nerve
C5/6	Arm abduction (deltoid), elbow flexion (biceps)	Axillary, radial	Biceps	Lateral arm, thumb and index finger	Cutaneous nerve of arm, musculocutaneous
C6/7	Wrist extension (extensor carpi radialis)	Radial	Brachioradialis	Lateral forearm, middle digit	Lateral antebrachaial cutaneous
C7/8	Elbow extension (triceps)	Radial	Triceps	Middle digit, medial hand	Median, radial
C8/T1	Grip (flexor digitorum profundus), finger abduction (interosseous)	Ulnar		Medial hand and forearm	Ulnar, medial cutaneous nerve
L2/3	Hip flexion (iliopsoas)	Femoral	Cremasteric	Anterior, superior thigh	Genitofemoral, femoral
L3/4	Knee extension (quadriceps)	Femoral	Patellar quadriceps	Mid medial thigh and calf	Obturator
L4/5	Ankle dorsiflexion (hamstrings, tibialis anterior)	Peroneal		Medial and anterior calf	Sural, dorsal cutaneous
L5/S1	Knee flexion (hamstring), foot inversion (posterior tibialis), great toe extension (extensor hallucis longus)	Peroneal, sciatic/ tibial nerve		Lateral calf and foot (medial L5, lateral S1)	Sural, dorsal cutaneous
S1/2	Ankle plantar flexion (gastrocnemius)	Sciatic/tibial nerve	Achilles gastrocnemius	Foot, posterior	Sural
S2-4	Rectal tone (bowel/bladder, anal sphincter)	Pudendal	Anal cutaneous, bulbocavernosus	Perianal area	Pudendal, coccygeal

ACUTE SPINAL CORD INJURY[9–11]

Epidemiology: 50/1 million per year

- M > F (mainly in adolescent males)
- 20% of patients with spinal cord injury have more than one level affected
- Major causes of death are aspiration and shock

Etiology: Fractures, dislocation, distraction, mass (tumor, epidural abscess, epidural hematoma, etc.), penetrating (knives, bullets, etc.), ischemic

COMPLETE

No residual function more than three levels below the injury

- Only 3% of patients will recover some function within 24 hours, after which the expectation is that all distal function is likely lost

INCOMPLETE

Any residual sensory or motor function below the injured level

- Sacral sparing: Sensation and voluntary rectal sphincter contraction (excluding sacral reflexes)
- Examples: Central cord syndrome, Brown-Séquard syndrome, anterior or posterior cord syndromes

Imaging: STAT MRI of affected levels, CT of entire spine to evaluate for additional fractures

Treatment: Prevent secondary injuries; ABCs; methylprednisolone protocol as established by the National Acute Spinal Cord Injury (NASCIS) randomized controlled trials remains controversial when considering benefits vs. complications associated with high-dose steroids

- Surgery emergently with progressive neurological deficits, otherwise operate in 1 to 2 weeks (also controversial) for spine stabilization

▧ Central Cord Syndrome

Usually an extension injury with underlying chronic cervical spondylosis where the central region of the spinal cord is injured

Symptoms:

- Disproportionately greater motor impairment in upper extremities than lower extremities (hand > upper extremities > lower extremity dysfunction), bladder dysfunction, variable sensory changes

▧ Brown-Séquard Syndrome

Spinal cord hemisection (e.g. knife assault)

- Ipsilateral weakness (descending motor fibers), loss of contralateral pain and temperature (spinothalamic tracts), loss of ipsilateral vibration and proprioception (dorsal columns)

Table 12-3 Frankel Grade and Muscle Strength Testing[12]

Muscle Strength Testing		Reflexes	
Score	Exam	Root Level	Reflex
0	No movement	C5	Biceps
1	Visible contraction	C6	Brachioradialis
2	Movement without gravity	C7	Triceps
3	Movement with gravity	L4	Knee jerk
4	Less than full strength	S1	Ankle jerk
5	Full strength		

Frankel Grade (ASIA)		Upper vs Lower Motor Lesions		
Grade	Function	Findings	UMN	LMN
A	Complete paralysis	Strength	↓	↓
B	Sensory function only below level of injury	Tone	↑	↓
C	Incomplete motor function (grade 1–2/5 below injury level)	Deep tendon reflex	↑	↓
D	Fair to good motor function (grade 3–4/5 below injury level)	Superficial tendon reflex	↓	↓
E	Normal function (5/5)	Babinski	+	−
		Clonus	+	−
		Fasciculations	−	+
		Atrophy	−	+

Lumbar Spinal Stenosis

Canal ≤ 12 mm
Stenosis ≤10 mm AP diameter
Lateral recess stenosis < 2 mm
UMN: Upper motor neurons; LMN: Lower motor neurons.

▮ Cauda Equina Syndrome

Neurosurgical emergency
- Injury to lumbosacral nerve roots

Symptoms: Motor/sensory deficits corresponding to affected nerve roots (severe radiculopathy or myelopathy), bowel or bladder incontinence, perineal numbness (late)

Signs: Pain out of proportion to exam, digital rectal exam with decreased rectal tone, abnormal postvoid residual (> 200 cc)

Etiology: Compressive lesion, usually from herniated disc, cancer, trauma, or infection

Radiology: STAT MRI of thoracic and lumbar spine (compression can be anywhere from conus down to sacral region and is usually central)

Treatment: Emergent surgical decompression

INDICATIONS AND CONTRAINDICATIONS FOR EMERGENT SPINE SURGERY[13]

Indications

1. Cauda equina syndrome
2. Acute, severe neurological deficit (e.g. myelopathy of vital cervical root) — controversial
3. Mechanical instability, usually secondary to trauma (e.g. nonreducible fracture-dislocation with locked facets)

Contraindications: Complete spinal cord injury > 24 hours (not absolute), medically unstable (e.g. uncorrectable coagulopathy, unstable angina)

INITIAL MANAGEMENT OF ACUTE SPINAL CORD INJURY (SCI)[14–16]

Follow ATLS protocol (airway, breathing, circulation, disability)

- Intubation may be necessary if diaphragm paralyzed (above C5) or altered level of consciousness
- Avoid neck extension and fibro-optically intubate if necessary
- Maintain oxygenation and blood pressure to ensure appropriate perfusion of spinal cord and to avoid exacerbation of injury
- Additional injuries below level of injury may be missed due to lack of signs/symptoms and fixed bradycardia/hypotension from loss of sympathetic tone
- Maintain immobilization and spine precautions until appropriate diagnostic procedures and evaluations can be undergone

■ Methylprednisolone Protocol (Controversial)

Must be administered within 8 hours of SCI (outcome may be worse if started after with increased risk of infection, ventilator dependence, and pneumonia)

- 30 mg/kg loading dose, 45 min pause, followed by 5.4 mg/kg for 23 hours (if started within 3 hours of injury) or 47 hours (if between 3–8 hours from surgery)

Table 12-4 NEXUS Criteria for Cervical Spine Imaging in Pediatric Blunt Trauma*

NEXUS criteria	Operator Characteristics**
Midline tenderness	95% confidence intervals (CI)
Impaired consciousness, poor history	Sensitivity 100% (89–100%, 95% CI)
Neurologic deficit	Specificity 20% (19–21%, 95% CI)
Distracting/painful injury	Negative PV 100% (99–100%. 95% CI)
Intoxication	Positive PV 1% (1–2%, 95% CI)

*NEXUS Cspine study included 3065 patients < 18 years old (88 < 2 years old, 817 - 2–8 years old, & 2160 - 8–17 years old). Criteria may not apply if < 2 years, trauma with underlying congenital/acquired spine instability (Down's, Juvenile rheumatoid arthritis syndrome, Klippel-Feil syndrome, prior fracture)
**PV – predictive value

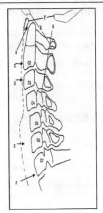

Figure 12-1 Normal Cervical Spine Spaces

A - Atlantal dens interval-(predental space) < 5mm if < 8 years, > 8 years < 3mm

B - Posterior cervical line, spino-laminar line of C2 should be within 2 mm anterior or posterior to line

C - Prevertebral space ≤ 7 mm in front of C2 or < 1/3 width of C2 vert. body

D - Limit of overriding of vertebral bodies is 2.5 mm

E - Retrotracheal space should be < 14 mm in front of C6 or < 5/4 of width of C5 in front of C5 (# are inexact)

F - Prevertebral fat stripe should not bulge out

X ÷ Y = Power's ratio

Normal value is 0.7 – 1.0

Value < 0.7 suggests anterior subluxation atlantooccipital (AA) joint. Also, a line from the anterior margin of the foramen magnum to the tip of the odontoid should be < 10–12 mm. If greater, atlantooccipital dislocation may be present

Wackenheim's line: a line drawn along posterior clivus usually intersects tip of odontoid tangentially. If displaced, suspect atlantooccipital joint laxity

May be unreliable in young children

▮ Neurogenic Shock[10]
Hypotension secondary to interruption of sympathetics (loss of vascular tone), bradycardia from unopposed parasympathetics, relative hypovolemia due to venous pooling from decreased muscle tone, and hypothermia
- Generally above the T6 level
- Treat hypotension with dopamine gtt (epinephrine can exacerbate bradycardia)

▮ Spinal Shock
Transient flaccid paralysis and areflexia after acute spinal cord injury, which transitions into spasticity in 1–2 weeks

ISCHEMIC SPINAL CORD INJURY

Etiology: Arterial or venous; atherosclerosis, diabetes, aortic aneurysms or dissection, sickle cell, trauma, arteritis, AV fistula, hypercoagulable state, hypotension

- Spinal cord has one anterior and two posterior spinal arteries
- Watershed area in mid-thoracic region is susceptible to ischemic injury in severe hypotension or vascular injury to the aorta
- Artery of Adamkiewicz leaves from around T9 and disruption may lead to anterior spinal syndrome
- Vertebral artery injury may lead to cervical cord ischemia from disruption of the posterior spinal arteries

Symptoms: Pain, weakness, paralysis, loss of sensation, incontinence

Treatment: Symptomatic, maintain blood pressure to increase spinal cord perfusion

ANTERIOR SPINAL ARTERY SYNDROME

Flaccid transitioning to spastic paralysis, hyperreflexia, loss of pain and temperature, intact vibratory and proprioception (posterior column function preserved)

TRAUMA[1,17–19]

5% of spinal column injuries involve multiple levels

CRANIO-CERVICAL MEASUREMENTS

▮ AtlantoOccipital Dislocation[23]
Severe hyperextension-distraction injury rupturing craniocervical ligaments (tectorial membrane, cruciate, apical, alar) and frequently resulting in fatal brain stem injury (respiratory arrest)
- Basion-dental interval (inferior tip of clivus to top of odontoid) > 12 mm
- More common in children

• May be atraumatic in Down syndrome, rheumatoid arthritis
Treatment: Cervical fusion (historically halo rigid immobilization)

▓ Clinical Criteria to Clear Cervical Spine
Awake, alert, oriented
• No neck pain, either to palpation or to active range of motion (flexion, extension, and lateral rotation)
• Not intoxicated
• No distracting injuries
• No focal neurological deficits

If patient cannot be clinically cleared, may require an MRI to rule out ligamentous injury. If patient has no evidence of fracture on a cervical spine CT, but does have tenderness to palpation or pain with range of motion, a flexion-extension film with view of C7 is indicated.

▓ AtlantoDental Interval (ADI)
Distance on lateral X-ray between back of C1 anterior tubercle (atlas) to the anterior aspect of the odontoid (dens)
• Normal for adult is up to 3 mm, in child is up to 5 mm (pseudosubluxation)

▓ Chamberlain's Line
Posterior aspect of hard palate to posterior edge of foramen magnum or opisthion
• If the dens is > 6mm above this line, consistent with vertical translocation

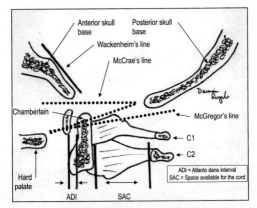

Figure 12-2 Atlantooccipital Axis Measurements

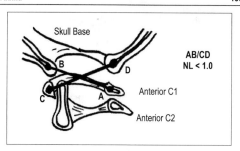

Figure 12-3 Power's Ratio

▓ Fischgold's Digastric Line
Between the digastric notches

▓ Fischgold's Bimastoid Line
Between tips of mastoid process

▓ McGregor's Line
Dorsal edge of the hard palate to the caudal occiput
- If dens is > 4.5 mm, consistent with invagination

▓ McRae's Line
Opening of the foramen magnum
- Tip of dens should not be above this line

▓ Power's Ratio
Identify anterior subluxation (see Figure 12-3)
- Ratio of BC (distance from the basion to the midvertical portion of the posterior laminar line of the atlas) over OA (opisthion to midvertical portion of posterior surface of anterior ring of atlas)
- Anterior subluxation present if ratio is > 1

▓ Ranawat's Line
Center of the C2 pedicle to a line connecting the anterior and posterior C1 arches
- < 13 mm designates impaction

▓ Redlund-Johnell Measurement
From base of C2 to McGregor's line
- Pathological when less than 34 mm in men and 29 mm in women
- Designates basilar invagination

▓ Rule of Spence
On odontoid view X-ray, if sum of C1 lateral mass overhang on C2 is 7 mm, then this suggests transverse ligament instability

▓ Wachenheim's Line
To determine subluxation
- Line from the posterior surface of the clivus to the odontoid tip
- Constant in flexion-extension
- Should not be > 5 mm

▓ Denis Three-Column Classification (for Thoracolumbar Fractures)
- Anterior column: Anterior 50% of vertebral body, disk, and anterior longitudinal ligament
- Middle column: Posterior 50% of vertebral body, disk, and posterior longitudinal ligament
- Posterior column: Pedicles, lamina, spinous processes (essentially all posterior elements)

ODONTOID FRACTURE[17]

Flexion or extension loading
- Transverse ligament must be intact for atlantoaxial stability and non-operative management
- Associated with atlas fracture (Jefferson fracture)
- Developmentally, ossification centers are two primary (inferiorly to either side of midline) and one secondary (apical)

▓ Rule of Thirds
Dens 1/3, spinal cord 1/3, empty 1/3

▓ Type I (Tip) (Figure 12-4)
Stable
- Avulsion of alar ligament insertion (connects dens to occiput)
- Treat with collar

▓ Type II (Base) (Figure 12-5)
Most common dens fracture
- Unstable due to disruption of blood supply
- Nonunion in up to 50%, especially in elderly, increased translation, or angulation
- Requires halo placement (younger, < 5 mm translation) or surgical management such as an odontoid screw or historically a C1–C2 posterior arthrodesis with wire (must have intact C1 posterior arch)

▓ Type III (Body) (Figure 12-6)
Stability depends upon degree of displacement, unless the fracture extends into facets
- Heals with immobilization— collar in elderly or if stable, otherwise halo; if no fusion, then anterior odontoid screw

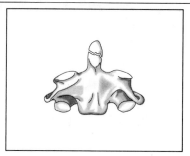

Figure 12-4 Type I Odontoid; Fracture (Stable)

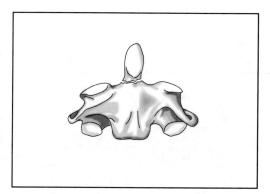

Figure 12-5 Type II Odontoid; Fracture (Unstable)

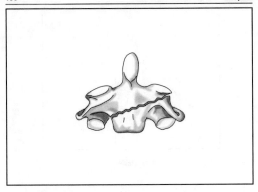

Figure 12-6 Type III Odontoid; Fracture (Stable)

■ Odontoid Screw Placement
Goal is anterior, inferior, midline endplate of C2 in midline
- Will maintain normal range of motion when compared to posterior fusion; may reduce the need for postoperative external orthosis immobilization (e.g., halo)

JEFFERSON'S FRACTURE (FIGURE 12-7)
- Comminuted C1 ring fracture (bilateral fracture of anterior and posterior arches)
- Most common fracture of C1
- Fracture from axial load of atlas via occipital condyles
- Neurological deficits rare, occasional injury to vertebral artery
- Treated with a hard collar if there is no disruption of the transverse atlantal ligament (TAL) and can be treated with halo or surgical fusion if TAL is disrupted
- If TAL is intact is determined by ADI and Rule of Spence (C1 separated by dens > 7 mm)

HANGMAN'S FRACTURE (FIGURE 12-8)
- Bilateral C2 pars/pedicle fracture with avulsion of C2/C3 endplates, slippage of C2 on C3; separation of posterior elements from the vertebral body
- The worse the angulation and slippage, the worse the grade

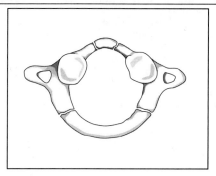

Figure 12-7 Jefferson Fracture of C1

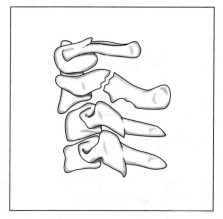

Figure 12-8 Hangman's Fracture

Table 12-5 Fracture Types and Columnar involvement

Type	Anterior	Middle	Posterior
Compression	Compression	None	None or distraction
Burst	Compression	Compression	None or distraction
Seat-belt	None or compression	Distraction	Distraction
Fracture/ dislocation	Compression ± rotation/shear	Distraction ± rotation/shear	Distraction ± rotation/shear

Stable Spine Fracture Criteria:	Gun Shot Wounds to the Spine (remove bullet/fragment - decompress):
-No transient or persistent neurological injury	-Progressive neurologic deficit due to neural compression (bullet, fragment, hematoma)
-Acceptable alignment	-Incomplete neurologic deficit
-At least 1 column intact	-High energy weapon (large internal zone of injury/damage along projectile tract)
-No significant ligamentous disruption	

Source: Spine, 8:1983.

- Mechanism: Hyperextension, compression (axial loading) and distraction
- May present with instant death due to spinal cord transection or no neurological deficits

Grade 1: Minimal distraction (< 3 mm), anterior longitudinal ligament (ALL) torn

- Stable, treat with collar

Grade 2: Moderate distraction/angulation (> 4 mm), ALL and posterior longitudinal ligament (PLL) torn, disk herniation

- Unstable, treat with halo

Grade 3: Significant distraction, torn ligamentous complex, epidural/spinal cord hematoma, locked facets, vertebral artery injury, disc herniation

- Flexion injury that may result in locked facets or subluxation of C2 on C3
- Unstable, treat with surgery

CERVICAL FACET DISLOCATION[25,26]

Pathophysiology: Flexion/rotation injury → unilateral, flexion/distraction → bilateral

- Disruption of the anterior and posterior longitudinal ligaments with facet articular capsule tears → sliding the superior facet forward on the inferior facet
- Superior vertebral body displaces anteriorly, disc may herniate posteriorly

Complications: Ipsilateral vertebral artery injury, posterior longitudinal ligament injury, canal stenosis, cord compression

Table 12-6 Cervical Spine

Injury/Eponym	Classification/Limits	Treatment
Occipital condyle fracture[28]	I - Impaction	Hard collar
	II - Plus skull fracture	Hard collar
	III - Avulsion	May require halo immobilization
Occiput-C1 dislocation	Anterior or posterior (usually fatal)	Halo & occiput/C1 fusion
C1 fracture[29] (Jefferson = axial load)	A. Transverse process	Stable fractures (posterior arch or nondisplaced fractures) treated with cervical orthosis
	B. Posterior arch	
	C. Anterior arch	Asymmetric lateral mass fracture or Jefferson "burst" fractures require halo immobilization
	D. Comminuted or lateral mass	
	E. Burst	Transverse ligament rupture without a bony avulsion requires fusion
Odontoid fracture[30]	I - Oblique apical/avulsion	Cervical orthosis (beware associated injury)
	II - Base fracture (high nonunion rate ~ 36%)	Halo vest, internal fixation for age > 50, > 5 mm, displaced posterior displacement, screw fixation vs. fusion
	III - Fracture into body	Halo immobilization

Traumatic spondylolisthesis[29] of C2 Hangman's fractures	I - Nondisplaced par (no angulation, < 3 mm)	Cervical orthosis
	II - Displaced/angulated	Reduction/halo
	IIa - C2–3 disc torn, anterior longitudinal ligament intact	Reduction/halo
	III - Fracture/ dislocation	Attempt reduction (< 4 mm translation, < 10° angulation) halo (failure: Rule out disc rupture, ± fusion)
C3–C7 Facet dislocation	Unilateral (< 25% displacement of vertebral body Bilateral (25–50% displacement of vertebral body)	Traction (10 lb + 5 lb/level), open reduction/posterior fusion failed closed reduction, consider MRI; rule out disc herniation
C3–C7 Fracture	Translation angular displacement	> 3.5 mm - fusion, > 11° - fusion
C3–C7 Burst	Canal compression	< 25% compression with intact posterior wall = nonoperative. Stable = Halo immobilization, unstable = fusion
C3–7 Spinous process fracture	Clay shoveler's fracture	Symptomatic

Source: Anderson/Montesano[28]; Levine/Edwards[23]; Anderson/ D'Alonzo[30]

- Bilateral facet injuries generally have corresponding complete spinal cord injury

Treatment: Posterior, posterior or combined cervical decompression, reduction and stabilization with or without discectomy

■ **Facet Orientation**[27]
- Cervical → posteromedial
- Upper thoracic → coronal (resistance to anterior translation but not rotation)
- Lower thoracic → sagittal (less resistance to anterior translation)

TEARDROP FRACTURE

Flexion-compression injury
- Vertebral body with > 50% original height
- Injury to the posterior longitudinal ligament
- Unstable

WEDGE FRACTURE

Fracture of the anterior column
- Stable if < 50% loss of height → can observe with brace

SPINOUS PROCESS FRACTURE

Are stable in isolation
- When occurring at C7, is referred to as a *clay-shoveler's fracture*

BURST FRACTURE (TABLE 12-7)

Fracture of the anterior and middle columns from axial compression injury
- Usually between T10 and L2
- Can be treated with brace or surgery depending on the complexity
- Surgery if greater than 50% canal compromise or greater than 50% vertebral body height loss or with facet fractures or dislocations
- May lead to retropulsion of bony fragments into the spinal canal with devastating neurological compromise

Table 12-7 Thoracic and Lumbar Spine

Burst fracture	A - Axial load B - Axial & flexion C - Axial & flexion D - Axial & rotation E - Axial & lateral flexion	Stable = hyperextension cast/brace Unstable (height < 50%, angulation > 20°, canal compromise > 50%, scoliosis > 10°, neurologic injury) = early operative stabilization
Flexion/ distraction Chance Fracture		Bony = hyperextension cast Soft tissue = Open Reduction Internal Fixation (ORIF)
Fracture -dislocation	Flexion – rotation Shear	ORIF - early mobilization

FRACTURE DISLOCATION

Disruption of the anterior, middle, and posterior columns
- Almost always requires surgery

CHANCE FRACTURE

A flexion-distraction fracture through all three spine columns (including disruption of PLL, shearing of pedicle/vertebral body)
- Dislocation of facet joint leading to a "naked" facet
- May have associated spinal cord injury or hematoma
- Usually in the thoracic spine of a person who had a lap belt on and was in a motor vehicle accident (MVA)
- Due to etiology of injury (e.g., severe MVA with seatbelt) up to 30% will have associated abdominal organ injury

SCHMORL'S NODES

Herniation of the nucleus pulposus into the end plate
- Associated with endplate fracture
- T7–L2

HALO PLACEMENT[31,32] (FIGURE 12–9)

Indication: Treatment of cervical spine trauma, preoperative reduction for spinal deformity, postoperative stabilization

Contraindications: Open wounds or infection at proposed pin sites, cranial fracture (relative contraindications include obesity, elderly, barrel-shaped chest, severe chest trauma)

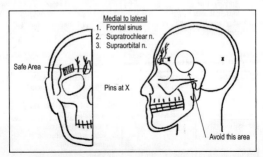

Figure 12-9 Halo Placement

Procedure:

1. Patient should be positioned on a spine board with the semirigid collar in place until the halo is intact
2. While stabilizing the spine, slide the back panel under the patient's back between the scapulae
3. Attach the occipital support to the back panel
4. Size the ring to ensure 1 cm clearance between the scalp and ring
5. Choose the pin insertion site as shown: just below maximum head circumference, just above eyebrows, and 1–2 cm above pinnea
6. Shave and sterilize area for pin insertion
7. Ensure adequate analgesia with low-dose fentanyl and local anesthetic with lidocaine injection
8. Ask patient to close eyes (avoid skin traction)
9. Tighten diagonally opposite pins simultaneously to finger tight, then 1 inch-pound at a time
10. Should end with 6–8 lb in for adults and 4–6 lb in for children. For children, be sure to measure skull thickness prior to placement; may also require up to eight pins
11. Tighten the locking nuts
12. Attach the halo to a vest
13. Retighten pins at 24–48 hours

Complications: Pin site infection, skull fracture, pin loosening, skin breakdown, inadequate healing requiring surgical intervention, pain, respiratory distress

TRACTION (GARDNER-WELLS TONGS) PLACEMENT[6,32,33]

Indication: Cervical spine instability, reduction of cervical deformity/jumped facets/fracture/dislocation in patient who will require surgical stabilization or nonhalo immobilization; may be used for temporary intraoperative stabilization

Contraindications: Resolving neurological symptoms, fracture requiring halo immobilization, depressed skull fracture, extensive distraction

Procedure: May be performed at the bedside or in the operating room prior to surgical stabilization

1. Provide adequate analgesia and muscle relaxation to allow for reduction
2. Position pins below the widest portion of the skull, below the temporal ridge, above the temporalis muscle, in line with the external acoustic meatus (above and anterior to the pinnea)
3. Place 1 cm anterior or posterior depending upon if flexion or extension is required for reduction (more anterior extends the neck, more posterior flexes)

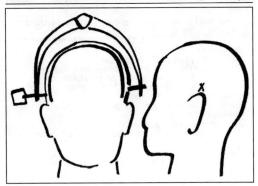

Figure 12-10 Gardner-Wells Tongs

4. Shave and sterilize area for pin insertion (optional)
5. Inject local anesthetic (lidocaine with epinephrine)
6. Apply Gardner-Wells tongs pins and screw into place, until indicator pin protrudes 1 mm (13.6 kg or 30 lb of pressure = 65–120 lbs of pull-out strength) (Figure 12–10)
7. Tighten the locking nuts
8. Incrementally apply weights to traction pulley (start with 5 lb; should not exceed 5 lbs for each level of injury, e.g., C5, 25 lbs)
9. Take lateral X-ray to confirm reduction
10. Ensure the knot does not drift up to the pulley, or else traction is not being applied

Complications: Dislodgement, inner table perforation, worsening of neurological injury, failed reduction, infection

DEGENERATIVE SPINE DISEASE

■ AtlantoAxial Impaction (Basilar Invagination) and Platybasia[24]
Subluxation of the dens (odontoid process) through the foramen magnum leading to brainstem compression

Symptoms: Myelopathy, headache, nystagmus, cranial neuropathies

Pathophysiology: Bony erosion between occiput and dens (e.g., rheumatoid arthritis); also associated with Chiari malformation, syringomyelia, Klippel-Feil syndrome

Treatment: Occiput to C2 fusion, possible transoral decompression

Radiculopathy: A nerve root or lower motor neuron (LMN) injury potentially causing unilateral dermatome pain and weakness as well as decreased reflexes

Myelopathy: A spinal cord or upper motor neuron (UMN) injury causing bilateral symptoms and can manifest as neck pain, weakness/numbness in extremities, hyperreflexia, gait instability, and urinary incontinence

Treatment: In the setting of nonurgent, stable disk herniations, nonoperative management should be tried for at least 2 months

- Natural history of many disk herniations, especially in the lumbar spine, is spontaneous resolution
- May undergo open or minimally invasive techniques for surgical removal of herniated disc
- Nonsurgical therapies: Rest, physical therapy, epidural steroid injections, selective nerve root blocks, acupuncture, radiofrequency ablation, intradiskal electrothermal treatment (IDET), chiropractic
- "Failed back syndrome" (patients with who have had multiple revision spine surgeries and have no clear pain generators at this point) may be treated by pain pumps and spinal cord stimulators

OSSIFICATION OF THE POSTERIOR LONGITUDINAL LIGAMENT (OPLL)

- Usually occurs in the cervical spine
- Segmental, continuous, or mixed
- Can be treated with laminectomy, laminoplasty, or corpectomy with instrumentation
- ACDF for this procedure frequently results in a CSF leak since the ligament is adherent to the dura
- Usually occurs on the posterior portion of the vertebral body in the cervical spine whereas ankylosing spondylitis (AS) has heterotopic ossification anterior and posterior to the vertebral body that can happen all along the spine

DISC HERNIATION

▓ Cervical Disk Herniation

Affects the nerve root of the lower vertebral body (e.g., C6 nerve root would be affected in a C5/C6 disk herniation, C8 nerve root affected in a C7/T1 disk)

- Most cervical disc herniations occur at C5/6, followed by C6/7
- Treat with anterior cervical decompression and fusion (ACDF) or if a posterolateral soft disc herniation, in singers or athletes, may do a posterior foraminotomy

▓ Thoracic Disk Herniation
Rare
- Most common at T11/12
- Should not be treated with laminectomy alone as risk for neurological injury or no improvement reaches 45%
- Approaches include transpedicular, transfacet, transthoracic or lateral extracavitary

▓ Lumbar Disk Herniation
Affects the nerve root of the lower vertebral body (e.g., L4 would be affected in an L3/4 central or paracentral disk herniation)

▓ Far-Lateral Disk Herniation
Will affect the nerve root of the higher vertebral body
- L3 would be affected in an L3/4 far-lateral disk herniation

SPINAL STENOSIS

SAC (space available for the cord) = spinal canal diameter

Central stenosis is a narrowing of the SAC from bone, disk, ligament, or foreign body encroachment

Foraminal stenosis is a narrowing of the neural foramen where the nerve root exits and can be bilateral or unilateral

SPONDYLOSIS[1,18]

Pathophysiology: Degenerative changes of the spine including facet hypertrophy, lamina and ligamentous hypertrophy, degeneration of the intervertebral disc, formation of osteophytes, autofusion of vertebral levels, and loss of cervical and lumbar lordosis

- Annular tears of the intervertebral disc occurs from collagen deposition, loss of water, and proteoglycan from the nucleus pulposus
- Spondylosis may lead to neural foramina narrowing, central spinal stenosis, decreased mobility, and kyphosis

Symptoms: Back pain, radicular pain, myelopathy

- In lumbar region can lead to neurogenic claudication, cauda equina syndrome

Treatment: Nonoperative management first → analgesics, anti-inflammatory, muscle relaxants, physical therapy, epidural steroid injections

- Cervical nerve root compression can be treated with dorsal foraminotomies
- Central cervical stenosis should be treated with anterior cervical decompression and fusion (ACDF)
- Lumbar central stenosis can be treated with decompressive laminectomies
- Lumbar radiculopathy can be treated with foraminotomy

LATERAL RECESS SYNDROME

Compression of nerve root in lateral recess between hypertrophied superior articular facet, pedicle, and inferior vertebral body
- Treat with laminectomy and medial facetectomy (1/3 of facet, more is destabilizing and may require fusion)

SPONDYLOLISTHESIS (FIGURES 12-11–12-15)

One vertebral body slips over another one
- Commonly in the lumbar spine (95% at L5) and is usually associated with bilateral pars interarticularis (spondylolysis) fractures but can be congenital, traumatic or degenerative
- Leads to foraminal stenosis commonly, but canal rarely compromised
- Pathologic process separates the spine into anterior (vertebral body, pedicles, transverse process, superior facet) and posterior (inferior facet, laminae, spinous process)

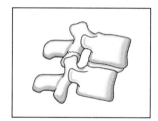

Figure 12-11 Grade I Spondylolisthesis (25%) Slippage

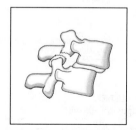

Figure 12-12 Grade II Spondylolisthesis (25-50%) Slippage

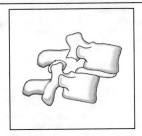

Figure 12-13 Grade III Spondylolisthesis (50-75%) Slippage

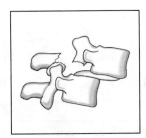

Figure 12-14 Grade IV Spondylolisthesis (75-100%) Slippage

- M > F
- Many spontaneously resolve, so treat conservatively first
- Indications for surgery include progressive spondylolisthesis, radiographic instability on flexion/extension films with corresponding mechanical pain, progressive neurological deficit or medically refractory pain

ISTHMIC SPONDYLOLISTHESIS

Abnormality of the pars interarticularis
- Degenerative (facet joint motion → intersegmental instability), traumatic (fracture of pedicle, articular processes), or pathologic (generalized disease process e.g., Paget's)

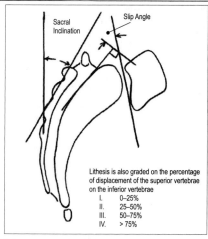

Lithesis is also graded on the percentage
of displacement of the superior vertebrae
on the inferior vertebrae

I.	0–25%
II.	25–50%
III.	50–75%
IV.	> 75%

Figure 12-15 Measurements in Spondylolisthesis

DYSPLASTIC SPONDYLOLISTHESIS

Usually L5–S1
- Facet joint subluxation

SPONDYLOPTOSIS

100% subluxation; synonymous with pars interarticularis defect or
fracture
- Occurs in up to 20% of the population

SURGICAL TREATMENT OPTIONS

See Operative Note Dictations Chapter 18 for further details

■ General Terminology

Laminectomy: Bilateral or unilateral removal of spinal lamina processes

Laminotomy: Partial removal of lamina to decompress or facilitate access to
a microdiskectomy

Diskectomy: Can refer to a partial or "microdiskectomy" or can be total removal
of disk material that may require a spacer and possible instrumentation

Table 12-8 Spondylolysis and Spondylolithesis

Class	Type	Age	Pathology/Other
I	Congenital	Child	Dysplastic S1 superior facet
II	Isthmic	5–50	Elongation/fracture of L5 S1 pars
III	Degenerative	*Older*	Subluxation due to facet (L4 L5) arthrosis Acute fracture (not pars)
IV	Traumatic	*Young*	
V	Pathologic	Any	Bony elements destroyed/incompetent
VI	Postsurgical	Adult	Over resected arches/facets

Lithesis Grades	
I.	0–25%
II.	25–50%
III.	50–75%
IV.	75–100%
V.	>100%

Spondylolysis
Defect in the pars interarticularis
Most common cause of low back pain in children
Fatigue fracture (gymnastics, football linemen)
80% visible on plain films, 15% on obliques (Scottie dog#)
Treatment is symptomatic, avoid extension
Casting for more severe or symptomatic cases

Foraminotomy: Decompression of an existing nerve root by removal of bone and ligament around the foramen

ISPD (interspinous process device): Sits between the spinous processes mechanically expanding the neural foramen at that level

■ Cervical Decompression and Fusion

Anterior Cervical Discectomy and Fusion/Foraminotomy (ACDF)

Indications: Persistent radiculopathy/myelopathy or neurologic deficit attributable to clear anterior pathology on MRI (e.g., single or two level herniated cervical disk), with normal spinal lordosis; destabilizing trauma

Outcome: Although the fusion rate for a single level ACDF is quite high (~95%) every level of surgery added increase the risk of nonunion. Surgeon preference dictates if a rigid collar is required or not

Complications: Injury to pharynx, esophagus, or trachea, vocal cord paresis (injury of recurrent laryngeal nerve/vagus; 11% temporary, 4% permanent[26]), vertebral artery, carotid artery, CSF leak, Horner's syndrome, injury to spinal cord/nerve root, inability to fuse, infection, and hematoma. Immobility at levels of fusion may increase stress on adjacent levels leading to progressive degenerative disease

■ Posterior Cervical Laminectomy +/- Fusion

Indications: For multiple cervical disc disease and myelopathy (with neutral or lordotic sagittal alignment), severe cervical stenosis with posterior compression, ossification of the posterior longitudinal ligament (OPLL), previous anterior approach, in individuals where risk of vocal cord paralysis is intolerable. This can be supplemented with lateral mass fusion

Lateral Mass Screw (Figure 12-16):

Magerl technique: Screw should be placed using an entry point 1 mm medial to dead center of the lateral mass and the trajectory should be to the upper outer quadrant to minimize vertebral artery and nerve root injury

Roy-Camille technique: Aiming "straight through" the lateral mass

Laminoplasty: An option that can be used in lieu of laminectomy/fusion, designed to preserve motion. Hinges one side of the posterior elements (lamina), then held open with instrumentation

Complications: Progressive kyphotic deformity, vertebral artery injury, CSF leak, injury to spinal cord/nerve root, inability to fuse, infection, and hematoma

■ Thoracic Fusion

The thoracic spine is technically challenging due to proximity of the cord, difficulty of access, critical vascular and pulmonary structures, and small pedicles for instrumentation. Thoracic laminectomy may need to include instrumentation (e.g., ankylosing spondylitis) as uninstrumented laminectomies for decompression may result in complete paraplegia

Approaches: Laminectomy, transpedicular, costotransversectomy, transthoracic

Complications: Radicular artery injury leading to spinal cord ischemia, pneumothorax, CSF-pleural fistula, pneumonia, vascular injury (aorta/vena cava), CSF leak, injury to spinal cord/nerve root, inability to fuse, infection, and hematoma

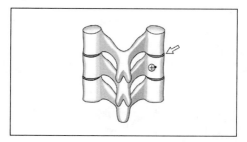

Figure 12-16 Trajectory for Lateral Mass Screw Placement

▇ Lumbar Fusion

Depending upon the approach, may involve laminectomy, discectomy, placement of bone graft, and instrumentation. A general rule about lumbar pedicle screw placement is that as you progress down the levels, you should "medialize" the screw trajectory between 15° and 30° (15° at L1 to 30° at L5). The entry point is usually at the transverse process/facet junction. Complications depend on the approach utilized, but generally include durotomy, neurological injury, infection, and implant migration. Caution in osteopenia/osteoporosis

Anterior Lumbar Interbody Fusion (ALIF)

Good for L5/S1 or revision cases where you do not want to go through a posterior approach (avoids removal of posterior musculature). Cannot decompress from this approach so must be combined with a posterior approach if stenosis present. At some institutions, the approach is performed by vascular or general surgery. Anterolateral approach is for L2–5 and is 30° lateral to the direct anterior approach (L5S1).

Complications include injury to abdominal vessels or bowel, ileus, retrograde ejaculation (so not done on young, male patients), abdominal hernia

Lateral Interbody Fusion

Tubular dilators are inserted via a flank incision, and EMG monitoring through the psoas helps to avoid nerve root injury. Generally restricted to levels L3–5 as one is limited caudally by the iliac crest and rostrally by the ribs

Unique complications: include psoas muscle weakness (generally transient), and injury to the nerves running on or through the psoas muscle

Posterior Lumbar Interbody Fusion (PLIF)

A full laminectomy and diskectomy is done with an interbody graft placed into the disk space from either side. This construct is then usually supplemented with pedicle screws. Can only be done at lower levels because requires significant retraction on the dural sac. Epineural fibrosis may lead to chronic radiculopathy

Transforaminal Lumbar Interbody Fusion (TLIF)

Similar to PLIF, but more lateral approach allows for less retraction on the Approach is from one side and the facet is taken down allowing access to the disk space for the diskectomy. A single banana-shaped interbody graph is slid across the midline and the construct is usually supplemented with pedicle screws. Puts greater tension on the nerve root so runs higher risk of neuropathy

SPINAL CORD TUMORS[8]

EXTRADURAL (55%)

Outside the spinal cord and dura (e.g., epidural or in the vertebral body)

- Frequently metastatic lesions in the adult and neuroblastoma or Ewing's sarcoma in kids

Metastatic

Lymphoma, lung, breast, prostate → destructive; prostate, breast → osteoblastic

Primary

Chordoma, neurofibroma, osteoid osteoma (benign, posterior lumbar spine, night pain improved with aspirin, lytic lesion with calcifications), osteoblastoma, aneurysmal bone cyst, chondrosarcoma, osteochondroma (benign but locally invasive, cervical spinous/transverse process), vertebral hemangioma, giant cell tumor of bone, osteosarcoma (malignant, osteolytic/sclerotic lesion on CT, survival < 1 year)

Miscellaneous

Plasmacytoma, multiple myeloma, eosinopholic granuloma, Ewing's sarcoma, chloroma, angiolipoma, hemangioendothelioma, giant cell tumor (benign but locally invasive, sacrum, lytic mass on CT)

Perineural (Tarlov) Cyst

Occurs at the junction of the dorsal nerve roots and ganglia most commonly at the sacrum

- Between the endoneurium and perineurium
- May present with pain (e.g., sciatica), urinary incontinence, sexual dysfunction, weakness
- Spontaneous rupture may lead to headache from intracranial hypotension from CSF leak from cyst
- F > M
- Treatment: Cyst drainage (usually recur), steroid injections, microsurgical resection

EOSINOPHILIC GRANULOMA

Lytic lesion without surrounding sclerosis

- Classic cause of single collapsed vertebral body in pediatric patient, if no evidence of trauma
- Bright on T2, enhances with contrast

ANEURYSMAL BONE CYSTS[37,38]

Epidemiology: Age less than 20

- Associated with eosinophilic granuloma, fibrous dysplasia, giant cell tumor
- Benign

Radiology: Posterior cervical, thoracic area

- CT shows a lytic lesion with surrounding cortical bone
- MRI shows lobulated fluid-fluid levels from blood degradation products

EPIDERMAL LIPOMATOSIS

Pathogenesis: Chronic hypercortisolemia, obesity, idiopathic

Presentation: Radicular, myelopathic symptoms of thoracic, lumbar region

Treatment: Conservative; weight loss, decreased steroid dose, decompressive laminotomy

INTRADURAL EXTRAMEDULLARY (40%)

In the nerve root or leptomeninges

▓ Schwannoma/Neurofibroma
Homogeneously enhancing dumbbell shaped tumor that extends through neural foramen; usually can spare the nerve in a schwannoma since the nerves do not run in the tumor as is the case with neurofibromas

▓ Meningioma
Classically well circumscribed, homogeneously enhancing; 15% are extradural

▓ Paraganglioma
Usually occurs in the cauda equina region

▓ Cysts
Arachnoid, dermoid/epidermoid, and neurenteric

▓ Lipoma

INTRAMEDULLARY (5%)

In the spinal cord
- 15% of primary CNS tumors are intraspinal[35]

▓ Ependymoma (40%)
Cellular type occurs in the cervical region whereas the myxopapillary type occurs at the conus. These can usually be separated out since there is often a well-defined plane between tumor and spinal cord. Goal is gross total resection.

▓ Astrocytoma (40%)
Most common intramedullary spinal cord tumor in children. Usually in the cervical region and can have an associated syrinx. These tumors are more difficult to get a gross total resection and may require postsurgical adjuvant therapy

▓ Miscellaneous (20%)
Includes, dermoid, epidermoid, teratoma, lipoma, hemangioblastoma, neuroma, lymphoma, oligodendroglioma, cholesteatoma, intramedullary metastases

Differential Diagnosis of a Cauda Equina Tumor

Myxopapillary Ependymoma, schwannoma, paraganglioma, meningioma, drop metastasis, lymphoma, hemangioblastoma (esp. with Von Hippel-Lindau)

SPINAL AVMS[1]

Present with progressive neuro deficits or a sudden onset of myelopathy secondary to hemorrhage

TYPE I

Dural AV fistula

- Extramedullary, no nidus, low flow, simple dorsal venous drainage, lower thoracic/conus
- Most common in adults (85% of spinal AVMs)
- Present with progressive neurological deficits secondary to venous congestion

Treatment: Coagulate feeder vessel as it enters nerve root sleeve versus embolize → curative

TYPE II

Glomus

- Intramedullary, may present with hemorrhage, high flow, cervicothoracic junction

Treatment: Surgical excision after embolization

TYPE III

Juvenile

- Intra- and extradural but with intramedullary nidus, high flow, cervical/upper thoracic
- Very rare, marked propensity to bleed, multiple feeders over multiple segments, present with progressive neurological deficit
- Prognosis poor, secondary to size, vascular complexity, and intervening normal spinal cord tissue

■ Type IV

Perimedullary dural AV fistula with extramedullary AVM nidus

- Progressive neurological deterioration

Treatment: Coagulate vessel as it enters nerve root sleeve versus embolize versus radiosurgery; trap nidus feeder vessels with temporary clips and check for neuromonitoring changes before cauterizing permanently

Subtypes: I (single feeder, low flow), II (multiple feeders, increased venous engorgement), III (giant, multiple feeders, high flow, vascular steal)

FOIX-ALAJOUANINE SYNDROME[38]

Thrombosis of spinal cord AVM

Location: Lower thoracic, lumbar, sacral

Pathology: Necrosis of gray > white matter

Presentation: Subacute myelopathy

SYRINGOMYELIA

A syrinx or intramedullary cavity formation within the spinal cord (distance from the central canal) that fills with CSF (see Table 12-9)
- Syrinx can be associated with Chiari malformation, trauma, spinal cord tumor, or anything affecting flow of CSF through the spinal cord
- Can treat syrinx with shunt or midline myelotomy, but it's best to try to remove the source of the syrinx

Symptoms: Transient pain, dissociated sensory loss (loss of pain and temperature) in upper extremities, motor disturbances, spastic paraparesis; may lead to neuropathic arthropathy = charcot or neurotrophic joint (loss of proprioception and deep sensation leads to recurrent trauma to and destruction of the joint); if in the cervical region can lead to respiratory compromise

SYRINGOBULBIA

Syrinx extends into the medulla
- Symptoms include those of syringomyelia but also include bulbar signs (weakness of tongue, pharynx, larynx)

HYDROMYELIA

Dilation of the central canal
- Has ependymal lining
- Etiology: Congenital, postraumatic, tumor

TRANSVERSE MYELITIS

Sudden onset of autoimmune demyelination or inflammation across one spinal cord segment

Etiology: Lupus, postinfectious viral or bacterial, vaccinations, Behçet's, idiopathic, multiple sclerosis

Presentation: Sensory level, weakness, pain, paralysis, urinary incontinence

DDx: Infarct, lymphoma, multiple sclerosis

Workup: CSF cytology and protein, multiple sclerosis panel, MRI brain and full spine

Treatment: Steroids

SUBACUTE COMBINED DEGENERATION[18]

Symmetric spinal cord demyelination from B_{12} deficiency

Etiology: B_{12} deficiency from pernicious anemia

Symptoms: Lower extremity paresthesias, sensory loss, spastic paraparesis, ataxia, confusion, dementia, peripheral neuropathy, megaloblastic anemia

Pathology: Wallerian degeneration

- Vacuolar disturbance of myelin sheath
- Cervical, thoracic > lumbar
- Posterior columns, spinocerebellar tracts, corticospinal tracts

VITAMIN E DEFICIENCY[39]

Ataxia, decreased reflexes, acanthocytosis, hemolytic anemia, peripheral neuropathy, spinocerebellar tract degeneration, weakness, loss of proprioception and vibratory sense

PEDIATRIC SPINE (TABLES 12-9–12-11)

OS ODONTOIDEUM[40]

Absent, hypoplastic, or unfused dens
- May be a congenital lack of fusion but generally considered to be post-traumatic
- Generally stable and incidentally found
- May present with neck pain
- No edema and ossified margins differentiate it from an acute fracture

KLIPPEL-FEIL SYNDROME[41,42]

Congenital fusion of two or more cervical vertebrae (usually involves C2–3)

Etiology: Associated with mutation on chromosome 8

- Failure of cervical vertebral (somite) segmentation

Grading:

- Type I: Fusion of cervical and upper thoracic vertebra with synostosis
- Type II: Isolated cervical spine fusion
- Type III: Cervical vertebra associated with lower thoracic or upper lumbar fusion

Table 12-9 Cervical Spine Anatomy in Children < 8 Years Old

- Normal lordosis to cervical spine is absent in 14% of children
- Normal posterior angulation of odontoid seen in up to 4% of children
- Majority of injuries occur at C1-C2 ≤ 8 years old and lower cervical spine > 8 years
- Os odontoideum: Congenital anomaly where odontoid does not fuse with C2*
- Ossiculum terminale: A secondary center of ossification for odontoid tip, appears by age 3 (in 26% of children) and fuses with odontoid by 12 (may never fuse)
- Prevertebral space at C3 is ≤ 1/3–2/3 of C3 vertebral body width or ≤ 5–7 mm
- Prevertebral space at C5 is ≤ 5/4 of (C5 or C6) vertebral body width or ≤ 14 mm**
- Predental space up to 5 mm ≤ 8 years (up to 3 mm > 8 years)
- Pseudo-Jeffersonian fx: C1 lateral masses grow faster than C2 so C1 overlaps C2 (usually < 6 mm). Present in 90% age 1–2, 18% aged 7 years
- Pseudosubluxation of C2/C3 or C3/C4 in 40% (normal variant where anterior aspect of C2 spinolaminar line is ≤ 2 mm ant or post to posterior cervical line

*Spine injury with minor trauma occurs, **These norms can be unreliable in children

Table 12-10 Development of Cervical Spine

Age	Feature
< 6 mo	C1 body invisible and all synchondroses are open, vertebrate are normally wedged anteriorly, and there is often no lordosis to the noninjured spine
1 yr	Body of C1 becomes visible radiographically
3 yr	Posteriorly located spinous process synchondroses fuse, dens becomes ossified (visible radiographically)
3–6 yr	Neurocentral (body) and C2-odontoid synchondroses fuse
	Summit ossification center appears at the apex (top) of the odontoid
	Anterior wedging of the vertebral bodies resolve (and is not normal if seen)
8 yr	Pseudosubluxation and predental widening resolve, lordosis is normal now
12–14 yr	Secondary ossification centers appear at spinous process tips, summit
	Ossification center of odontoid fuses (if it does no to os odontoideum occurs), superior/inferior epiphyseal rings appear on body
25 yr	Secondary ossification centers at tips of spinous processes fuse, superior/inferior epiphyseal rings fuse to vertebral body

Source: Used with permission Tarascon Pediatric Emergency Pocketbook, 4th ed. Tarascon Publishing, Lompoc, CA[43]

Table 12-11 Pediatric Spine Ossification Center Fusion

Age (years)	Fusion Of
2–3	Neural arch posteriorly
3–6	Body of C2 with odontoid process*
7	Anterior arch with neural arch

*This fusion line (subdental synchondrosis), or the remnant of the cartilaginous synchondrosis, can be seen until age 11 years and may be confused with a fracture
Source: Lustrin[32]

Symptoms/Signs: Short/webbed neck, decreased cervical spine range of motion, low hairline

- May be incidental, or with torticollis, neck webbing, facial asymmetry

Associations (up to 70%): Sprengel's deformity (congenital elevation of scapula, occurs in 30%), Chiari I, scoliosis, spina bifida, basilar impression, genitourinary, cranial, facial, and cardiac abnormalities

- Can lead to traumatic quadriplegia after minor trauma

Treatment: Medical management of multiple comorbidities

- For spinal instability external immobilization (halo) versus surgical fusion

PEDIATRIC SPINAL CORD INJURIES

Children are more likely to have ligamentous injury rather than bony fractures, due to relatively large size of head and ligamentous laxity

- Synchondroses may be mistaken for fracture line, pseudospread of the atlas misdiagnosed for a Jefferson fracture, and pseudosubluxation

Epidemiology: Rare (< 5% of SCI occur in children), tend to involve the cervical spine, higher fatality rate than with adults

- More susceptible to spinal cord injury without radiologic abnormality (SCIWORA)

SPINAL CORD INJURY WITHOUT RADIOLOGIC ABNORMALITY (SCIWORA)[43–45]

Epidemiology: 1/5 of all pediatric spinal cord injuries

- > 80% involve cervical cord
- Most occur and are the most severe in children < 8 years old

Pathophysiology: Pediatric spine is inherently elastic, permitting self-reduction but severe intersegmental displacement

Imaging: Immediate CT normal, MRI normal in 50%

- Delayed MRI shows spinal cord atrophy

Symptoms/Signs: Pure sensory 44%, pure motor 31%, mixed 25%

Treatment: Supportive care, steroid treatment (controversial), bracing may not be necessary

Prognosis: May recover if initial MRI is negative

- > 50% have delayed onset of neurological deficit (may have paresthesias at time of accident), which is rapid and may lead to a complete lesion

SPINE GLOSSARY

Sagittal balance: Global balance of the head, cervical, thoracic, lumbar spine and pelvis on sagittal view when the patient is standing with his or her knees straight. Best assessed with 36" standing scoliosis films

Cantilever forces: A beam supported on only one end that allows for overhanging structures without external bracing. An example would be the forces experienced by a pedicle screw from the attached rod construct

Posterior tension band—Stabilizing forces in the posterior elements that inhibit forward flexion. Usually ligamentous forces and can be simulated with posterior wiring techniques in case of disruption.

Pull-out strength—Intrinsic resistance to a screw or screw construct from backing out of the bone. This is usually enhanced by "medializing" or "lateralizing" the screw trajectory and adding a cross-link to make it a solid wedge of bone between the screws.

Three-point bending—Term applied usually to a construct involving three adjacent vertebral bodies where the middle one is misaligned and the flanking ones allow for support to pull it back. Usually in cases of spondylolisthesis.

Glacial instability—Similar to global vertebral body instability that can result in mechanical or axial back pain.

Anterior column reconstruction—Important when trying to regain normal lordosis for kyphotic deformity correction. Usually requires an anterior approach.

Axial loading—Downward forces applied to the spine along its axis. Can be chronic, acute, or traumatic. Traumatic axial loading can result in spine fractures such as a Jefferson's C1 ring fracture.

Dynamic stabilization—Spine instrumentation that allow for some preservation of motion such as an artificial disk, load sharing rods, etc.

Ligamentotaxis—This is when spine constructs are used to manipulate bone structures in such a way as to move bone that is attached to ligaments. An example would be pedicle screw distraction of a lumbar burst fracture to move the retropulsed fragment out of the canal.

CHAPTER 13 ■ NEUROVASCULAR

Anthony Wang, MD
Melanie G. Hayden Gephart, MD, MAS

ANEURYSMS[1,2]

Epidemiology: Prevalence up to 5% in general population

- Incidence increases with age
- F > M
- 15–30% of patients have multiple aneurysms
- Yearly risk of subarachnoid hemorrhage (SAH) approximately 1–2%/year in incidentally discovered aneurysm (see Table 13-1)

Types: Saccular (most common), fusiform, dissecting

Source: Embolic (infectious), traumatic, inflammatory, neoplastic, radiation-induced, congenital predisposition, atherosclerotic, flow related (e.g., arterio-venous malformation [AVM]), or hypertension

- Saccular aneurysms are acquired lesions from degeneration of the internal elastic lamina, defects in the muscularis media

Risk factors: Bacterial endocarditis (streptococcal), coarctation of the aorta, Osler-Weber-Rendu, fibromuscular dysplasia, AD polycystic kidney disease, AV malformation, Ehlers-Danlos, pseudoxanthoma elasticum, familial intracranial aneurysm syndrome are diseases associated with aneurysm formation

Location: Branch points of major cerebral arteries likely saccular aneurysm. Saccular 85–95% anterior circulation (ACoA most common), 5–15% in posterior circulation

- Distal aneurysms more likely from traumatic or mycotic source
- Mycotic aneurysms commonly in middle cerebral artery distribution
- Traumatic aneurysms occur on the distal anterior cerebral artery due to shearing injury against the falx
- Fusiform aneurysms are more likely in the vertebrobasilar system
- Location may determine symptoms; for example, with posterior communicating aneurysm → 3rd nerve palsy

Symptoms of SAH: Headache, nausea, vomiting, meningismus, photophobia, confusion, loss of consciousness, coma

- "Worst headache of life"
- May have a "sentinel bleed" resulting in headache, dizziness, up to a week before major SAH

Table 13-1 Presentation

Major Rupture	Comments	Other Signs
Subarachnoid hemorrhage	Most common	Sentinel hemorrhage, headache
Intracerebral hemorrhage	20–40%, usually major cerebral artery	Mass effect
Intraventricular hemorrhage	Worse prognosis (especially with increased ventricular size)	Hydrocephalus

Table 13-2 Potential Localizing Signs in Intracerebral Hemorrhage of Aneurysmal Etiology

Aneurysmal Intracerebral Hemorrhage	
Location	Possible Localizing Signs
Acom	BLE weakness, numbness
MCA bifurcation	Contralateral weakness, aphasia (left), or hemi-neglect (right)
Basilar tip	Vertical ophthalmoplegia
Vertebral-PICA junction	Wallenberg's, vertigo, Horner's, sensory deficits
ICA-Pcom junction	Ipsilateral CN III palsy (pupil involving)

Table 13-3 Fisher Grading System

Fisher Grade	CT Subarachnoid Hemorrhage
1	None
2	Diffuse, thin layer (< 1 mm)
3	Localized clot or thick layer (> 1 mm)
4	Thin or no SAH along with ICH or IVH

Sources: Fisher[3], Claassen et al[4]

Fisher and associates[3] correlated the location and thickness of subarachnoid blood on CT with clinical outcome and likelihood of developing vasospasm. The Fisher CT grade (Table 13-3) is commonly used with the Hunt and Hess grade to gauge the severity of SAH

Treatment: Medical management (blood pressure control, stool softeners, calcium channel blockers and bed rest), surgical clipping of the aneurysm versus endovascular coils placed to thrombose the aneurysmal sac

- Treatment choice controversial, however, coiling helpful if the lesion is surgically inaccessible, or if the patient is elderly (> 75 with decreased morbidity with coiling) or with multiple co-morbidities; good neck-dome ratio

Outcome: Risk of repeat hemorrhage after aneurysmal SAH highest in first 2 weeks

Table 13-4 Hunt-Hess Subarachnoid Hemorrhage Grading System

Grade	Symptoms
1	Asymptomatic or mild headache and slight nuchal rigidity
2	Moderate to severe headache, nuchal rigidity, or cranial nerve palsy (CN III,VI)
3	Lethargy, confusion, or mild focal deficit
4	Stupor, moderate to severe hemiparesis, or early decerebrate rigidity
5	Coma, decerebrate rigidity, moribund appearance

Source: Hunt[5]

Table 13-5 5-Year Cumulative Rupture Rates (%) According to the Size and Location of the Unruptured Aneurysm

	< 7mm	7–12 mm	13–24 mm	25 mm
Cavernous Carotid	0	0	3.0	6.4
Anterior Circulation	0*	2.6	14.5	40.0
Posterior Circulation	2.5*	14.5	18.4	50.0

*If SAH occurs from a different aneurysm, risk increases 0.9–1.5
Anterior Circulation includes anterior cerebral, middle cerebral, internal carotid
Posterior Circulation includes basilar, posterior cerebral, posterior communicating
Source: White[7]

- 50% of untreated, ruptured aneurysms hemorrhage within first 6 months, then drops to 3%/year
- Mortality much higher in repeat SAH than the first hemorrhage

CEREBRAL VASOSPASM

Generally occurs following subarachnoid hemorrhage (SAH) from ruptured aneurysm (very rare in trauma) (see Table 13-5)
- May be clinical (symptomatic neurologic deficit) or radiographic

Incidence (following SAH): Clinical up to 30%, radiographic up to 70%[9]

- Onset between days 4–14 post-SAH, most frequently during days 6–8[10]
- Risk of clinical vasospasm increases with Hunt-Hess grade from 1 (22%) to 5 (74%)[11]

Symptoms: Depend on distribution of vasospasm (e.g., anterior cerebral artery (ACA) has frontal lobe findings, leg weakness)

DDx: Infection, hydrocephalus, seizure, cerebral edema, rehemorrhage, electrolyte disturbance (e.g., hyponatremia), hypoxia

Diagnostic Studies: Rule out other causes of neurologic deterioration (head CT to rule out hydrocephalus, CSF studies to rule out infection, EEG to rule out seizure)

- Transcranial Dopplers may have increased mean middle cerebral artery (MCA) velocity with an increased MCA:ICA (Lindegaard) ratio; levels

Table 13-6 Risk of Vasospasm

Modified Fisher	CT Appearance	Risk (%)
1	Thin subarachnoid hemorrhage	10
2	Bilateral intraventricular hemorrhage (IVH)	20
3	Thick cisternal clot	20
4	Bilateral IVH + cisternal clot	40

Source: Frontera et al[6]

above 120 cm/sec (ratio > 3) or daily increases of > 50 suggest vasospasm; Lindegaard ratio distinguishes vasospasm from hyperemia
- Angiogram for diagnosis and treatment

Treatment: Calcium channel blocker (e.g., nimodipine), hyperdynamic aka "triple H" therapy (hemodilution, hypertension, hypervolemia; for secured aneurysm), balloon angioplasty, intra-arterial injection of antispasmodics, intravascular stent

Prognosis: Most significant cause of morbidity (7%) and mortality (7%) from ischemic infarct in patients who survive initial SAH[9,11]

ARTERIOVENOUS MALFORMATIONS (AVM)[8,9]

Pathology: Congenital dilated communication between the arterial system and the venous system without capillaries

- AVMs are mid-high pressure systems with high flow rates
- Progressive neurological deficit may result from "steal" phenomenon where blood flow is diverted to AVM from normal brain parenchyma

Epidemiology: Average age of diagnosis is 33 yrs

- Risk of bleeding is 2–4% per year
- Usual presentation is hemorrhage
- Increased risk of hemorrhage in pregnancy

Radiology: Can be diagnosed via CT, MRI, or angiography

- 10% associated with flow dependent, intranidal aneurysm

Treatment: Endovascular embolization followed by surgical excision

- Stereotactic radiosurgery (indicated for deep lesions < 2.5 cm; requires 1–3 yrs for ablation during which hemorrhage rate is 2–3%/yr)
- General rule: Grade 1–3 AVMs can be operated on with an acceptable risk of complications (compared to the natural history of untreated AVM)

Table 13-7 Spetzler-Martin AVM Grading System

Characteristics	Comments	Points
Size	Small (< 3 cm)	1
	Medium (3–6 cm)	2
	Large (> 6 cm)	3
Eloquence of nearby brain tissue	Noneloquent	0
	Eloquent	1
Venous drainage pattern	Superficial only	0
	Deep	1

Grade = size, eloquence, and drainage scores added together
Source: Spetzler[9]

Table 13-8 Surgical Outcome and Spetzler-Martin AVM Grading System

Spetzler-Martin AVM Grade	No Deficit (%)	Minor Deficit (%)	Major Deficit (%)
1	100	0	0
2	95	5	0
3	84	12	4
4	73	20	7
5	69	19	12

Source: Spetzler[9]

- Patients with a score of greater than 3 have a high risk of complication and many surgeons recommend nonsurgical management
- Postoperative complication of normal perfusion pressure breakthrough necessitates tight blood pressure control (usually mean arterial pressure 60–80 overnight) to avoid hemorrhage and edema

Outcome: 10% mortality and 30–50% morbidity with each hemorrhage

DURAL ARTERIOVENOUS FISTULA[10–12]

AVM involving the dura

- Anomalous connection between the pial/dural arteries and the dural venous sinus

Epidemiology: 10–15% of all AVMs

- 66% in females age 40–50 years
- May result from trauma
- Commonly present with tinnitus
- Increased risk of hemorrhage with retrograde cortical venous drainage

Location: Most commonly seen at the lateral (transverse) sinus (L > R) at the junction of the lateral sinus with the sigmoid sinus

Treatment: Embolization (transarterial or transvenous), surgery, or stereotactic radiosurgery

- Indicated if neurological dysfunction, hemorrhage, or refractory symptoms or if retrograde cortical venous drainage discovered

Outcome: Hemorrhage → morbidity/mortality of 30%

CAROTID CAVERNOUS FISTULA

May lead to increased intraorbital pressure (from optic congestion) and resulting blindness

- Transvenous embolization treatment via inferior petrosal sinus can be curative

Epidemiology: 10–15% of all AVMs

- 66% in females age 40–50 years
- May result from trauma
- Common signs/symptoms present with tinnitus, bruit, headache, visual impairment, papilledema
- Increased risk of hemorrhage with retrograde cortical venous drainage

VENOUS MALFORMATIONS (AKA DEVELOPMENTAL VENOUS ANOMALIES)[13,14]

Low flow, low pressure systems

Epidemiology: Up to 2% of the population

- May be associated with cavernous malformations (30%), sinus pericranii, cortical dysplasias
- Multiple in Blue rubber bleb nevus syndrome
- Rarely if ever bleed (bleeding usually due to associated AVM or cavernous hemangioma)

Presentation: Most are incidental

- Rarely result in seizures or hemorrhages

Pathophysiology: Benign, developmental venous drainage of normal brain (deep white matter)

- Dilated anomalous veins or dilation of normal veins, which drain to transcortical vein

Location: Occur anywhere

- Supratentorial hemispheric white matter

Treatment: Rarely required

Radiology: Seen as starburst or "caput medusae" patterns on angiography

Outcome: Generally do not cause symptoms or require treatment

- Thrombosis may lead to a venous infarct because these anomalous veins drain normal brain tissue

CEREBRAL VENOUS SINUS THROMBOSIS[14–17]

Etiologies: Dehydration (esp. in infants from nausea/vomiting), diabetes mellitus (especially with ketoacidosis), infection (usually local, e.g., mastoiditis), pregnancy and puerperium (highest risk in first 2 wks after birth), birth control pills, homocystinuria, Behçet's syndrome, cardiac disease, ulcerative colitis, sickle cell trait, closed head injury, iatrogenic (radical neck surgery, transvenous pacer, postcraniotomy), periarteritis nodosa, malignancy, hypercoagulable state, and rarely lumbar puncture

Symptoms/Signs: Headache, nausea, vomiting, seizures, hemiparesis, cranial nerve dysfunction, papilledema, blurred vision, altered mental status

Diagnosis: CT ("delta sign" looking at sagittal sinus), MRI with MRV, angiography (for therapeutic intervention)

Treatment: Aggressive heparin anticoagulation to recover ischemic tissues (monitoring for the heightened risk of hemorrhage), +/− thrombolytics, correct underlying disorder, avoid steroids, control blood pressure, monitor ICP (lower ICP increases coagulability), intravascular stenting

VERTEBRAL ARTERY DISSECTION[18–21]

Presentation: Acute onset of neurological deficit

- Occipital neck pain, severe headache, altered mental status, SAH, TIA/ stroke (usually lateral medullary syndrome), cerebellar infarction, neck hematoma, embolic stroke

Spontaneous origin: Due to oral contraceptives, fibromuscular dysplasia, Marfan's syndrome, Moyamoya, cystic medial necrosis, Ehlers-Danlos, Takayasu's disease, and migraines

- Common in young males
- Commonly occur on the dominant vertebral
- 36% with other dissections present, 21% have bilateral vertebral dissections

Traumatic origin: Secondary to minor neck/posterior head trauma (chiropractor, MVA, sudden head turning) or sporting activity

- C1–C2 subluxation
- May lead to pseudoaneurysm development

Treatment: Anticoagulation or antiplatelet therapy for 6 months

- If SAH, symptoms despite medical therapy, progressing dissections, or intradural dissection, surgery, or interventional treatment (angioplasty and/or stent) may be indicated

INTERNAL CAROTID ARTERY STENOSIS [22,23]

Pathophysiology: Atherosclerosis of the common carotid artery

Presentation: TIA or acute neurological deficit

- Amaurosis fugax, blindness, MCA symptoms (such as contralateral arm/face motor/sensory deficits with hyperreflexia), and language deficits

Radiology: Duplex ultrasound (but cannot scan above the mandible), CT angiogram, angiography (expensive, invasive, and risky), or MRA (can overestimate the degree of stenosis)

Treatment: Antiplatelet therapy, blood pressure, and lipid control

- Intraarterial stenting
- Carotid endarterectomy (CEA) is helpful for stenosis 60–80% depending upon surgical risk and symptoms
- Complications of CEA include stroke, hemorrhage, vocal cord paralysis, hypoglossal nerve injury, mandibular nerve injury, bleeding, infection, seizures, and recurrent stenosis

CAVERNOUS HEMANGIOMA (AKA CAVERNOUS MALFORMATION, CAVERNOMA) [24]

Low flow, low pressure vascular malformations

Epidemiology: Majority are sporadic

- Familial inheritance autosomal dominant (AD) often in Latinos on chromosome 7 (KRIT1, MGC4607, PDCD10—role in angiogenesis)

Presentation: Seizures (60%), progressive neurological deficit (50%), and hemorrhage (20%), or hydrocephalus

- Most are asymptomatic

Location: Most supratentorial, but 10–23% in the posterior fossa around the pons

Radiology: Not easily seen on angiography but can be seen on MRI (flow void/previous hemorrhage) and CT (calcification or lucency)

- GRE is the most sensitive (for hemorrhage)
- Many have multiple lesions (> 20% with DVA)
- Well circumscribed
- May have associated AVM or venous malformation
- Enhances with contrast
- T2 may have a dark rim from hemosiderin deposition

Pathology: Irregular vasculature with no intervening brain

- "Popcorn" or "mulberry" appearance

Treatment: Controversial—observation, surgery for symptomatic/assessable lesions, and radiosurgery might be helpful to reduce the risk of rebleeding with inaccessible malformations

- Brainstem cavernous malformations should only be surgically resected if they have recurrent hemorrhage, reach a pial surface, and are symptomatic

Outcome: 0.25–0.75%/year untreated hemorrhage

- Hemorrhagic infratentorial lesions have increased risk of recurrent hemorrhage

MOYAMOYA DISEASE[25–27]

Epidemiology: Higher incidence in Japan than United States

- 0.9/100,000 in US

Symptoms/Signs: Seizures, hemorrhage, TIAs, stroke, progressive neurological deficit, cognitive decline

Pathophysiology: Progressive occlusion of one or both supraclinoid internal carotid arteries, M1 MCAs and A1 ACAs (and rarely P1 PCAs) resulting in a "puff of smoke" appearance of dilated capillary lenticulostriate collateral vessels

- Associated with intracranial aneurysms

Radiology: Angiography or flow voids seen on MRA

Treatment: Urgent decompression can be used if a patient presents with mass effect from hemorrhage

- Revascularization for those presenting with signs of ischemia, previous hemorrhage, or progressive neurological deficits can be performed on a nonemergent basis
- No medical or surgical treatment to date reduces rate of hemorrhage in Moyamoya disease
- Nevertheless, treating the patient for Moyamoya decreases the 5-year rate of stroke or death from approximately 65% to 5.5–17%
- Antiplatelet therapy, aspirin

AMYLOID ANGIOPATHY[28–30]

Epidemiology: Presents as lobar intraparenchymal hemorrhage (15% of ICH) in normotension, dementia

- Elderly

Location: Frontoparietal, corticomedullary junction

Radiology: GRE may reveal a higher number of hemosiderin depositions or "microbleeds"

Pathology: Deposition of beta amyloid in the media and adventitia of small and mid-sized arteries

- Primary amyloid (secondary in diabetes, beta microglobulinemia)

Treatment: Surgical evacuation may be considered in intermediate-sized hematomas (20–60 mL) with progressive deterioration in level of consciousness

Outcome: Hemorrhage recurrence rate of 38% with mortality rate of 44%

SYNDROMES WITH CEREBROVASCULAR DISEASE[31–32]

HEREDITARY HEMORRHAGIC TELANGIECTASIA (OSLER-WEBER-RENDU DISEASE)

Arteriovenous malformations of liver, lungs, brain, spine

Genetics: AD

- Mutation in TGF-beta receptor gene

Symptoms/Signs: In addition to AVMs, patients develop telangiectasias of skin, mucosa → epistaxis

- Nail bed telangiectasias, pulmonary shunt (high risk of brain abscess), cerebral aneurysms

WYBURN-MASON SYNDROME (AKA BONNET-DECHAUME-BLANC)

Multiple intracranial AVMs along the visual pathways (including optic tracts, midbrain) AVMs (including retina) and facial cutaneous vascular nevi

Symptoms/Signs: Optic nerve atrophy, seizures, strokes, subarachnoid hemorrhage

BLUE RUBBER BLEB NEVUS SYNDROME

Vascular malformations of skin, gastrointestinal tract, CNS (hemangiomas, venous angiomas, sinus pericranii)

Symptoms/Signs: Anemia from GI bleeds, nevi on arms/trunk/palms, fractures (from bone hemangiomas)

CHAPTER 14 ■ CRANIAL TRAUMA[1,2]

Melanie G. Hayden Gephart, MD, MAS

CLOSED HEAD INJURY[3-5]

Etiology: Primary (contusions, concussions, etc.) versus secondary (hypoxia, hypotension)

- Cerebral hypoxia → ATP depletion → failure of Na+/K+ pump → intracellular accumulation of Na+ and Ca+2 → acidosis, decreased NT uptake → glycolysis inhibition, increased extracellular glutamate → activation of NMDA channel → increased intracellular Ca+2 → protease/phospholipase activation → free fatty acid (free radical accumulation)
- Impairment of autoregulation of cerebral blood flow, decoupling of cerebral metabolism and cerebral blood flow

MONRO-KELLIE HYPOTHESIS

Brain parenchyma, blood, cerebrospinal fluid (CSF) in fixed box (skull)
- With increasing intracranial pressure (ICP), CSF production decreases, CSF is pushed into the spinal compartment, and resorption increases → intracranial blood volume decreased by venous compression → compliance decreases and small increases in volume lead to exponentially higher increases in ICP → eventually this culminates in brain parenchyma herniation, occlusion of arterial supply with resulting infarcts (see Herniation Syndromes, Chapter 20)

CEREBRAL EDEMA

Disruption of blood-brain barrier (vasogenic) or primary intracellular edema (cytotoxic)

CEREBRAL PERFUSION PRESSURE (CPP)

Normal 50 mmHg, should be > 60 mmHg in traumatic brain injury (TBI) patients
- CPP = MAP – ICP

MALIGNANT CEREBRAL EDEMA

In pediatrics with severe hyperemia, refractory increases in ICP, high morbidity/mortality
- Many have electrolyte, endocrine, and cardiopulmonary function abnormalities

TREATMENT CONSIDERATIONS FOR SEVERE HEAD TRAUMA

Neurological: Frequent neuro exams (q1hr), ICP monitoring device for GCS<8, prophylactic anticonvulsant therapy, consideration of evacuation of symptomatic mass lesions or hemicraniectomy.

Cardiovascular: Maintain systolic blood pressure > 90 < 160 (depending on baseline blood pressure and ICP), place arterial line and central line

Pulmonary: Intubation (for GCS < 8; inability to maintain adequate ventilation, impending airway loss from neck or pharyngeal injury, poor airway protection associated with depressed level of consciousness, and/or the potential for neurological deterioration)

Gastrointestinal: Stomach ulcer prophylaxis (e.g. proton pump inhibitor)

Genitourinary: Place Foley catheter (monitor urine output)

Hematologic: Check CBC, type and cross

Infectious disease: Consider antibiotic prophylaxis if a bolt or EVD is in place; tetanus, hemophilus, pneumococcus vaccine if indicated

Fluids/electrolytes/nutrition: NPO, isotonic saline (0.9% NaCl) with goal of euvolemia, check electrolytes, mannitol to temporize elevated ICP for refractory intracranial hypertension (to be held for serum osm > 320), hypertonic saline (goal of Na > 145)

Musculoskeletal: Ensure adequate tertiary survey, maintain cervical spine precautions until appropriately cleared

Disposition: ICU

MANAGEMENT OF CLOSED HEAD INJURIES IN PEDIATRICS

Table 14-1 Management of Closed Head Injury (CHI) in Children ≥ 2 Years Old

Inclusion Criteria[*]	Exclusion Criteria[**]
• Age 2-20 years • Normal mental status upon exam • Normal neurologic examination • May have LOC < 1 min, vomiting, headache, or lethargy which resolved • Evaluation within 24 hours of injury	• Age < 2 years • Signs of skull fracture • Multiple trauma or spine injury • Unobserved loss of consciousness • Bleeding diathesis underlying neuro. disorder (e.g., shunt, AVM)
Summary of American Academy of Pediatrics Recommendations	
Minor CHI, No LOC	• Observation in home, clinic, office, or ED • CT, MRI, and skull radiography are not indicated
Minor CHI, brief LOC *(Asymptomatic)*	• Option 1 – observation (home, clinic, office, ED, hospital) • Option 2 – CT is acceptable
Minor CHI, brief LOC *(Symptomatic)*	• Signs of CHI (e.g., lethargy, repeat vomiting, ↑ headache) • CT scan

[*]Inclusion and exclusion criteria for use of parameter.
[**]Does not imply mandatory imaging.
Source: *Pediatrics* 1999; 104: 1407.

CONCUSSION[6]

Definition: traumatic biomechanical force to the brain leading to short-lived impairment of neurologic function which resolves spontaneously. No abnormality on standard neuroimaging studies.

Signs and symptoms: somatic, cognitive, emotional, loss of consciousness, amnesia, behavioral changes, altered level of consciousness

Evaluation: remove from play and initiation of standard medical evaluation and exclusion of cervical spine injury. Assessment of concussive injury, followed by continuous observation and re-evaluation. **No return to play on the day of injury or while symptomatic.**

Graduated return to play protocol: Stepwise increase in activity (Table 14-2). If the patient is asymptomatic at the current level, may advance to the next level. If symptoms recurr, the player/patient should return to the prior asymptomatic level for at least 24 hours before attempting to increase activity.

Table 14-2

Graduated Return to Play (Objective)	Example
No activity (Recovery)	Complete rest
Light exercise up to 70% of MPHR (Increase HR)	Walking, stationary cycling
Sport-specific (Increase movement)	Drills, no contact
Non-contact training (Increase activity, coordination, cognitive demands)	Complex training drills
Full contact practice*	Normal training
Return to play	Competitive play, no restrictions
Modified from McCrory[6] *following medical clearance; MPHR - maximum predicted heart rate	

SKULL FRACTURES[3,5,7]

Diagnosis: Imaging (CT scan)

Radiology: Contre coup injury in 30% of cases

Treatment: Surgical debridement when wound is open, has greater than 0.5 cm of depression, or is cosmetically deforming

- Increased surgical risk if fracture is over a dural sinus
- Antibiotics may be indicated for open fracture

SIGNS OF SKULL BASE FRACTURES

Raccoon eyes (bilateral periorbital ecchymoses), mastoid ecchymoses, otorrhea/rhinorrhea of CSF, hemotympanum, cranial nerve palsy

- If concern for CSF leak, beta-2 transferrin is unique to CSF (and vitreous of the eye), but many times is a send-out lab that can take up to 1 week to return

TEMPORAL BONE FRACTURE

Longitudinal: more frequent (70–90% of temporal bone fractures) → facial nerve paralysis, hearing loss, vertigo, temporal/parietal trauma, epidural hematoma

Transverse: less frequent (10–30% of temporal bone fractures) → sensorineural hearing loss, equilibrium disorders, facial nerve injury

- Facial nerve damage more likely with transverse fracture, but overall longitudinal fractures are more frequent, so most facial nerve palsies are caused by longitudinal fractures

GROWING SKULL FRACTURE

Children (usually < 3 yrs) with fracture and underlying dural laceration, may result in progressive diastatic fracture and underlying leptomeningeal cyst

- Requires surgical intervention with repair of underlying dural defect

DIFFUSE AXONAL INJURY (DAI)

Etiology: Centripetal progression of neuronal disconnection (shear injury) secondary to severe, oblique vector (e.g. high-speed motor vehicle accident)
Clinical: Low GCS without obvious lesion on CT scan
Location: Corpus callosum, internal capsule, midbrain (tectum), basal ganglia, descending corticospinal fibers (pontomedullary junction)
Radiology: Punctate hemorrhages on MRI (GRE sequence most sensitive)
Outcome: Poor

EPIDURAL HEMATOMA

Radiology: 70% temporoparietal, 90% with fractures and underlying middle meningeal artery injury

- Lenticular, convex shape
- May have delayed enlargement
- Rarely associated with other brain injury (in comparison to acute subdural hematoma)

Outcome: 5% mortality , 10–30% delayed enlargement

Presentation: Most have history of severe head trauma

- Classically have a "lucid interval" with resolving confusion after initial injury and then neurological decline (actually occurs in < 30%)

Treatment: Surgical evacuation versus observation (if small and asymptomatic)

VENOUS EPIDURAL HEMATOMA

More frequent in children

- Next to the dural sinuses or tentorium

SUBDURAL HEMATOMA

Epidemiology: Occurs in 15% of severe head trauma

- Chronic subdurals are often seen in elderly with minor trauma especially when on anticoagulation
- Predisposition with conditions that cause brain atrophy and therefore, increased tension on bridging veins (e.g. alcohol abuse, dementia)

Etiology: Shear injury to bridging cortical veins (e.g., trauma, intracranial hypotension, severe atrophy, birth trauma)

Radiology (CT):

- Acute → hyperintense (can be isointense with low hematocrit or rapidly expanding lesions)
- Subacute → isodense
- Chronic (> 3 wks) → hypodense

Treatment: Patients with symptomatic SDH with midline shift should be surgically evacuated

- Acute SDH requires a trauma craniotomy; chronic SDH may be amenable to evacuation with burr holes

Outcome: 35–90% mortality, depending on chronicity, patient age, and comorbidities

- Reaccumulation of chronic SDH occurs in up to 45%

PENETRATING INJURIES[3,5,8]

Etiology: e.g., stab wound, gunshot wounds (GSW)

- Direct and indirect (temporary cavitation) injury
- Pressure waves lead to stretch injury in adjacent brain with high-velocity projectiles (e.g., GSW)

Radiology: CT scan. May see skull fragments, projectile debris

Treatment: Consider surgery for GCS 3–5 w/large EDH, GCS 6–8 without transventricular or bihemispheric injury, or GCS 9–15

Outcome: Mortality 70–80%

- 2/3 of victims die at the scene
- Post-traumatic epilepsy in 50% of survivors. If comatose at the time of presentation, mortality is > 90%

CHAPTER 15 ■ PERIPHERAL NERVES[1,2]

David McCall, MD

INTRODUCTION

There are three types of peripheral nerves: motor, sensory, and autonomic. Sensory nerve damage often results in tingling, numbness, pain, and extreme sensitivity in the distribution of the affected nerve. Motor nerve damage can lead to muscle atrophy, cramps, and spasms. Autonomic nerves control involuntary or semivoluntary functions, such as heart rate, blood pressure, digestion, and sweating. When autonomic nerves are damaged, this may lead to symptoms such as autonomic dysregulation, increased or decreased sweating, difficulty swallowing, nausea, vomiting, diarrhea or constipation, urinary dysfunction, abnormal pupil size, and sexual dysfunction.

PERIPHERAL NERVE INJURY AND HEALING

WALLERIAN DEGENERATION

Process of axonal degeneration distal to the site of injury or transaction; occurs in both the central and peripheral nervous system; injury → macrophages enter the axon and remove myelin/debris → Schwann cells stimulate axonal sprouts → axonal sprouts follow the basement membrane to the renewed connection → Schwann cells remyelinate the axon. Growth occurs at a rate of about 1 mm per day (= 1 inch per month and up to twice this rate in young children and infants).

- Muscles of mastication: All innervated by V3 of trigeminal nerve (CN V)
- Close jaw: Masseter, teMporalis, Medial pterygoid (M's Munch)
- Open jaw: Lateral pterygoid (L Lowers)
- Muscles of facial expression: All innervated by facial nerve (CN VII)
- Branches of the facial nerve (CN VII): "To Zanzibar by Motor Car": Temporal, zygomatic, buccal, masseteric, cervical
- Muscles with GLOSSUS: All innervated by hypoglossal (CN XII) except palatoglossus
- Muscles with PALAT: All innervated by vagus (CN X) except tensor veli palatini (V3 of CN V)

Table 15-1 Nerve Injury Classification

Seddon	Sunderland	Pathologic Findings
Neuropraxia	1	Localized myelin damage (compression)
Axonotmesis	2	Loss of axonal continuity; endo-, peri-, and epineurium intact
	3	Axonal and endoneurial continuity lost
	4	Axonal, endoneurial, perineurial continuity lost
Neurotmesis	5	Complete nerve lesion

Sources: Sunderland S. *Nerve injuries on their repair: A critical appraisal.* New York: Churchill Livingstone, 1991. Seddon HJ. *Surgical disorders of the peripheral nerves.* Baltimore: Williams and Wilkins, 1972, pp 68-88.

Number	Name	Foramen
I	Olfactory n	Olfactory foramina
II	Optic n	Optic canal
III	Oculomotor n	Superior orbital fissure
IV	Trochlear n	Superior orbital fissure
V	Trigeminal n	Superior orbital fissure, foramen rotundum, foramen ovale
VI	Abducens n	Superior orbital fissure
VII	Facial n	Stylomastoid foramen
VIII	Vestibulocochlear n	Internal acoustic canal
IX	Glossopharyngeal n	Jugular foramen
X	Vagus n	Jugular foramen
XI	Spinal accessory n	Jugular foramen
XII	Hypoglossal n	Hypoglossal canal

Figure 15-1 Cranial nerve number, name and exiting foramen

CERVICAL PLEXUS

From C1–C4 ventral primary rami

■ Motor branches

Ansa cervicalis
- Superior ramus (C1): geniohyoid and thyrohyoid muscles
- Inferior ramus (C2,3): SOS—sternohyoid, omohyoid, and sternothyroid
- Phrenic nerve (C3, 4, 5): "Keeps the Diaphragm Alive"

Sensory Branches
Lesser occipital, greater auricular, transverse cervical, supraclavicular, and meningeal branch that passes through foramen magnum

BRACHIAL PLEXUS

Randy Travis Drinks Cold Beer: roots (or rami), trunks, divisions, cords, branches

Roots: C5 to T1 ventral primary rami of spinal nerves

Trunks: Upper (C5, C6), middle (C7), and lower (C8, T1)

- Upper trunk yields suprascapular nerve (to supraspinatus and infraspinatus)

Divisions: Trunks split into anterior (3) and posterior divisions (3)

Cords: Lateral (upper and middle anterior divisions), medial (lower anterior division), and posterior (three posterior divisions)

- Lateral cord gives lateral pectoral nerve to pectoralis major
- Medial cord gives medial pectoral nerve to pectoralis major and minor and to the medial cutaneous nerve to the arm and the medial cutaneous nerve to the forearm
- Posterior cord: Upper (to subscapularis) and lower (to subscapularis and teres major) subscapular nerves and thoracodorsal nerve (to latissimus dorsi)

INJURIES TO THE BRACHIAL PLEXUS

Proximal Root Avulsion
Secondary to trauma → Horner's syndrome, phrenic nerve palsy

Long Thoracic Nerve Injury
Winging of scapula; need to be careful to identify nerve during lymph node dissection following mastectomy

Erb-Duchenne Palsy
Injury to upper trunk (C5,6) due to violent stretch between head and shoulder (commonly following shoulder dystocia) → affects dorsal scapula, suprascapular, lateral pectoral, long thoracic, musculocutaneous, radial, median, and phrenic nerves; loss of sensation in the radial side of the arm and hand, paralysis and atrophy of the deltoid, the biceps, and the brachialis muscles

- The arm hangs adducted and medially rotated with the elbow extended, forearm pronated (aka "Waiter's tip")

Klumpke's Palsy
Lower trunk injury to sudden pull upward of arm (birth palsy or from catching oneself from a fall) → loss of function of muscles of the hand and wrist

Axillary Nerve Injury
Caused by fracture of humeral neck or arm dislocation → paralysis of deltoid prevents arm abduction, lateral rotation of arm weakened

Table 15-2 Innervation of the Upper Extremity

Branch	From Cord	Motor Innervation	Cutaneous Innervation
Musculo-cutaneous	Lateral	Biceps, brachialis, coracobrachialis	Becomes lateral cutaneous nerve to forearm
Median	Lateral and medial	Pronator teres, flexor carpi radialis, palmaris longus, flexor digitorum superficialis, abductor pollicis brevis, supinator head of flexor pollicis brevis, oppones pollicis, 1st and 2nd lumbrical muscles	Radial 3½ fingers
Ulnar	Medial	Flexor carpi ulnaris, flexor digitorum profundus (3rd and 4th), palmaris brevis, abductor digiti minimi, oppones digiti minimi, flexor digiti minimi, 3rd and 4th lumbrical muscles, interossei, adductor pollicis, deep head of flexor pollicis brevis	Ulnar 1½ fingers
Radial	Posterior	Triceps, brachialis, brachioradialis, extensor carpi radialis longus and brevis	Posterior and lateral arm, back of hand up to nails
Axillary	Posterior	Deltoid, teres minor	Skin over deltoid
Posterior interosseous nerve	Posterior	Supinator, extensor carpi ulnaris, extensor digitorum, extensor digiti minimi, extensor pollicis longus and brevis, abductor pollicis longus, extensor indicis proprius	
Anterior interosseous nerve		Flexor digitorum profundus (1st and 2nd), flexor pollicis longus, pronator quadratus	

Table 15-3 Thumb Innervation and Action

Action	Nerve	Nerve Root	Muscle
ABduction (in plane of palm)	Radial	C7, C8	Abductor pollicis longus
ADduction (in plane of palm)	Ulnar	C8, T1	Adductor pollicis
ABduction (perpendicular to palm)	Median	C8, T1	Abductor pollicis brevis
Opposition	Median	C8, T1	Opponens pollicis
Flexion	Median	C8, T1	Flexor pollicis longus

Radial Nerve Injury
Wrist drop
  • Caused by midshaft humerus fractures

Median Nerve Injury
Ape hand (flattening of thenar eminence), thumb movement lost
  • Caused by supracondylar fractures, slashing of wrist, or carpal tunnel syndrome

Ulnar Nerve Injury
Claw hand
  • Can be caused by fracture of medial epicondyle of humerus or slashing of the wrist

FRACTURES OF THE UPPER EXTREMITY AND ASSOCIATED NERVE INJURY (TABLES 15-2 AND 15-3)

  • Surgical neck of humerus → axillary nerve
  • Midshaft fracture of humerus → radial nerve
  • Supracondylar fracture of humerus → brachial artery or median nerve
  • Medial humeral epicondyle fractures → ulnar nerve
  • Distal radius fractures → increase in carpal tunnel pressure and a median nerve compression

LUMBOSACRAL PLEXUS

  • Roots come from the ventral rami of spinal nerves L1–L5 and S1–S4 and a little of T12
  • Roots divide into anterior (ventral) and posterior (dorsal) divisions

LUMBAR PLEXUS (T12–L5)

  • Iliohypogastric (L1): Provides cutaneous innervation to hypogastric region
  • Ilioinguinal (L1): Cutaneous innervation to medial thigh and skin of external genitalia
  • Genitofemoral (L1,2 dorsal): Cutaneous to upper thigh and motor to cremaster muscle
  • Lateral femoral cutaneous (L2,3): Lateral cutaneous innervation of thigh

FEMORAL NERVE (L2,3,4 VENTRAL)

- Branches supply iliacus and psoas muscles in abdomen
- Cutaneous innervation of thigh down to the knee (except laterally)
- Supplies pectineus, sartorius, and four quadriceps muscles
- Provides articular innervation of the knee joint
- Terminates at the saphenous nerve; cutaneous to medial calf

Femoral Neuropathy

Cause: Thigh or pelvis trauma (hip, pelvis, or femur fracture, mass, ischemic nerve infarction or hip replacement, lithotomy position, diabetes mellitus)

Symptoms: Leg pain, quadriceps weakness, and sensory loss over thigh, and shin

Signs: Sensory loss, decreased patellar reflex

LATERAL FEMORAL CUTANEOUS NERVE (L2,3)

Innervates lateral thigh
- Compression leads to meralgia paresthetica

ACCESSORY OBTURATOR NERVE (L3,4)

Supplies pectineus and hip joint; only present in about 29% of people, obturator takes over function if absent

OBTURATOR NERVE (L2,3,4)

Supplies adductor magnus, longus, brevis, and gracilis muscles; also provides articular innervation to knee joint

LUMBOSACRAL TRUNK (L4,5)

Contributes to sacral plexus

SACRAL PLEXUS

SCIATIC NERVE (L4,5 S1,2,3)

- Tibial and common peroneal travel together as sciatic as far as the knee; divides into the tibial and common peroneal nerve at the superior border of the popliteal fossa
- Supplies hamstring muscles (biceps femoris [long head]), semitendinosus, Semimembranosus and adductor magnus muscles
- Has articular branches to the knee joint

Pudendal nerve (S3,4): Muscles of perineum and skin of external genitalia and anus

Nerve to quadratus femoris (L4,5, S1): Also supplies inferior gemellus

Nerve to obturator internus (L5, S1,2): Also supplies superior gemellus

Nerve to piriformis (S2, sometimes also S1)

Superior gluteal nerve (L4,5, S1): Supplies gluteus medius and minimus muscles and tensor fasciae latae

- Superior gluteal nerve injury leads to a positive Trendelenburg's sign (also seen with hip dislocations and femur neck fractures); contralateral pelvis drops when contralateral foot is raised

Inferior gluteal nerve (L5, S1,2): Supplies gluteus maximus

- Inferior gluteal nerve injury; can't sit up, climb stairs, or jump

Posterior femoral cutaneous nerve (S2,3 ventral; S1,2): Cutaneous innervation to buttocks and posterior thigh

▦ Sciatic Neuropathy

Causes: Trauma at sciatic notch or gluteal region (hip dislocation, fracture, or replacement), prolonged bed rest, deep-seated pelvic mass, piriformis syndrome (secondary to compression from sitting on one's wallet), tumor (schwannoma)

Symptoms: Lower leg pain and weakness

Signs: Sensory loss in peroneal, tibial, and sural territories, normal patellar reflex, femoral nerve normal

TIBIAL NERVE (L4,5, S1,2,3)

Supplies gastrocnemius, soleus, popliteus, plantaris, tibialis posterior, Flexor digitorum longus, and flexor hallucis longus; to posterolateral calf and foot
- Contributes medial component of sural nerve for cutaneous innervation
- Terminates as medial and lateral plantar nerves which supply muscles and cutaneous innervation of foot
- **TIP** = Tibial **I**nverts and **P**lantar flexes the foot

▦ Tibial Nerve Injury

Etiology: Trauma to popliteal fossa

Signs: Leads to calcaneovalgocavus, or dorsiflexion and eversion of foot

- Sensory deficit to the lateral and plantar surfaces of foot

COMMON PERONEAL NERVE (L4,5, S1,2)

- Innervates short head of biceps femoris in thigh
- Contributes lateral component of sural nerve; articular to knee joint

▦ Superficial Peroneal

Supplies peroneus longus and brevis and the skin over the dorsum of the foot

▦ Deep Peroneal

Supplies tibialis anterior, extensor digitorum longus and brevis, extensor hallucis longus, and peroneus tertius
- **PED** = **P**eroneal **E**verts and **D**orsiflexes (foot)

■ Peroneal Nerve Injury
Etiology: Trauma (including fibular head fracture), leg crossing

Signs: Lose dorsiflexion, sensory deficit on the dorsum of the foot especially between the big and second toe

LOWER EXTREMITY ANATOMICAL CONSIDERATIONS FOR PERIPHERAL NERVES (TABLES 15-4–15-5)

■ Popliteal Fossa
Diamond formed by hamstring muscles and two heads of gastrocnemius; contains tibial and common peroneal nerve, popliteal artery and vein, and small saphenous vein

■ Medial Malleolus Relationships
Anterior: Saphenous nerve and great saphenous vein (site for venous cutdown)

Posterior: **T**om, **D**ick, **A**Nd **H**arry: **T**ibialis posterior tendon, flexor **D**igitorum longus tendon, posterior tibial **A**rtery, tibial **N**erve, and flexor **H**allucis longus tendon

Table 15-4 Summary of Lower Extremity Innervation

Nerve	Plexus	Motor Innervation
Femoral	Lumbar	(Quadriceps femoris—rectus femoris, vastus lateralis, vastus medialis, vastus intermedius), iliacus, psoas, sartorius
Obturator	Lumbar	Adductor brevis, adductor longus, adductor magnus (along with tibial nerve), gracilis
Superior gluteal	Sacral	Gluteus medius, gluteus minimus, tensor facia lata
Inferior gluteal	Sacral	Gluteus maximus
Sciatic	Sacral	Semitendonosis, semimembranous, biceps femoris (long head [tibial division]), adductor magnus (with obturator nerve)
Tibial	Sacral	Gastrocnemius, soleus, tibialis posterior, flexor digitorum longus, flexor hallucis longus, medial and lateral plantar nerve
Deep peroneal	Sacral	Tibialis anterior, extensor digitorum longus, extensor hallucis longus, tibialis posterior, extensor digitorum brevis
Superficial peroneal	Sacral	Peroneus longus and brevis

DERMATOMES

C2	Back of head
C3	Turtleneck
C4	Polo collar
C5	Clavicle
C6	Thumb
C7	Middle and index fingers (radial nerve)
C8	Ring and little fingers (ulnar nerve)
T4	Nipple
T7	Xiphoid
T10	Umbilicus
T12	Inguinal region
L1–L4	Anterior and medial leg
L4	Big toe
L5	Dorsum of foot
S1	Plantar surface of foot and little toe, posterior calf
S2–S4	Perineum peripheral nerves

ENTRAPMENT SYNDROMES

OCCIPITAL NEURALGIA

Symptoms: Headache involving the posterior occiput in the greater or lesser occipital nerve distribution

- Pain in the neck, temple, and throbbing pain behind the eye on the ipsilateral side

Causes: Trauma or compression to the greater and/or lesser occipital nerves or C2 and/or C3 nerve roots by degenerative cervical spine changes, cervical disc disease, or tumors affecting the C2 and C3 nerve roots

Treatment: Occipital nerve decompression or stimulation

THORACIC OUTLET (SCALENUS ANTICUS) SYNDROME

Cause: Compression of subclavian vein or artery or brachial plexus between first rib and scalene muscles

- Also seen with cervical ribs
- Typically affects lower brachial plexus, C8–T1

Symptoms: Worsen with overhead activity

- May have edema and discoloration from venous congestion
- May have claudication symptoms from arterial compression

Signs:

- Adson's maneuver: Patient is asked to turn head toward the symptomatic shoulder while extending their arm, neck, and shoulder slightly

Table 15-5 Peripheral Nerves

Root	Nerve	Disc	Muscles	Weakness	Reflex
C4	Spinal accessory	C3–4	Trapezius, scalenus	Shoulder shrug	
C5	Axillary Musculocutaneous Radial	C4–5	Deltoid Biceps Brachioradialis	Shoulder abduction and external rotation, elbow flexion	Biceps, brachioradialis
C6	Axillary Musculocutaneous Radial	C5–6	Deltoid Biceps Triceps, brachioradialis, pronator teres, extensor carpi radialis	Elbow flexion, arm pronation, wrist and finger extension	Biceps, brachioradialis
C7	Radial Posterior interosseus Median Anterior interosseus Ulnar	C6–7	Triceps, pronator teres Extensor digitorum Flexor carpi radialis Flexor digitorum profundus 1 & 2 Flexor carpi ulnaris, flexor digitorum profundus 3 & 4	Elbow extension, wrist and finger extension	Triceps
C8	Radial Posterior interosseus Median Anterior interosseus Ulnar	C7–T1	Triceps Extensor digitorum Abductor pollicis brevis, opponens pollicis Flexor digitorum profundus 1 & 2 Flexor carpi ulnaris, flexor digitorum profundus 3 & 4, interossei, abductor digiti minimi	Finger flexion and abduction	Finger flexor

		Nerve	Muscles	Action	Reflex
T1	T1–2	Median Ulnar	Abductor pollicis brevis, opponens pollicis Flexor carpi ulnaris, flexor digitorum profundus 3 & 4, Interossei, abductor digiti minimi	Finger flexion and abduction	
L2	L1–2	Femoral Obturator	Iliopsoas, quadriceps Adductors	Hip flexion	Cremaster
L3	L2–3	Femoral Obturator	Iliopsoas, quadriceps Adductors	Thigh adduction, hip flexion	Knee
L4	L3–4	Femoral Obturator Superior gluteal Deep peroneal	Iliopsoas, quadriceps Adductors, sartorius Gluteus medius/minimus Tibialis anterior, extensor digitorum	Knee extension, ankle dorsiflexion and inversion	Knee
L5	L4–5	Superior gluteal Inferior gluteal Sciatic Tibial Medial/lateral plantar Deep peroneal	Gluteus medius/minimus Gluteus maximus Hamstrings Soleus, gastrocnemius, flexor digitorum Interossei Tibialis anterior, extensor digitorum	Thigh adduction and internal rotation, knee flexion, ankle and toe plantar and dorsiflexion	
S1	L5–S1	Superior gluteal Inferior gluteal Sciatic Tibial Medial/lateral plantar	Gluteus medius/minimus Gluteus maximus Hamstrings Soleus, Gastrocnemius, Flexor digitorum Interossei	Hip extension, knee flexion, ankle and toe plantar flexion	Ankle
S2	S1–2	Inferior gluteal Sciatic Medial/lateral plantar	Gluteus maximus Hamstrings Interossei	Toe cupping and fanning	

away from their body. The pulse on the wrist of the extended arm is checked while the patient inhales. If the pulse is diminished or symptoms are reproduced during the maneuver, it is considered a positive test result, which may indicate thoracic outlet syndrome. Repeat the test on the unaffected side

- Wright test: From a sitting position the arm is held back (hyperabduction), rotating it outward, while the pulse is checked to see if it's diminished
- Roos stress test: From a sitting position, the patient holds both elbows at shoulder height while pushing the shoulders back. The patient repeatedly opens and closes their hands for several minutes. A positive test occurs if symptoms are present after the test, or if heaviness and fatigue is felt in the shoulders
- Gilliatt-Sumner hand: Severe wasting of thenar and intrinsic muscles or the hand. Usually neurogenic in nature.

Treatment: Physical therapy, NSAIDs, resection of cervical rib

CARPAL TUNNEL SYNDROME (MEDIAN NERVE ENTRAPMENT AT WRIST)

Most common form of median nerve palsy

- F > M
- Intrinsic or extrinsic compression of median nerve in the carpal tunnel formed by flexor retinaculum over palmar surface of carpal bones
- Contents of the carpel tunnel: Flexor digitorum superficialis and profundus tendons, flexor pollicis longus tendon, and the median nerve
- Most common cause is overuse (e.g., computer typing, musicians)

Symptoms: Painful paraesthesia in distribution of median nerve (radial side of palm and 3.5 fingers)

- Burning feeling
- May radiate above wrist
- Common complaint is waking up with symptoms that are then relieved by shaking hands
- Decreasing grip strength

Signs:

- *Phalen's sign:* 90° flexion of wrist produces paresthesia
- *Tinel's sign:* Tapping of carpal ligament causes median nerve paresthesias
- Delay in palmar sensory conduction time is the most sensitive test

Treatment: NSAID, wrist splinting, corticosteroid injection, carpal tunnel release surgery

Ligament of Struthers (between distal humerus and medial epicondyle): Entrapment of the median nerve here leads to distal median nerve symptoms plus decreased pronation, wrist/digit flexion, thumb flexion, abduction, opposition

ULNAR NERVE ENTRAPMENT[3]

Most commonly elbow (cubital tunnel between the two heads of the flexor carpi ulnaris = most common); rarely at the wrist (Guyon's canal) or arm (Arcade of Struthers = aponeurosis anterior to the triceps band in the upper arm)

- Cubital tunnel syndrome is distinguished from compression in Guyon's canal by the presence of dorsal sensory deficits (absent in wrist compression)
- Will see motor deficits of ulnar distribution including adductor pollicis, deep head of flexor pollicis brevis, 3rd and 4th lumbricals, and sensory deficits in palmar surface of hypothenar eminence

Signs: Atrophy of hypothenar eminence and hand intrinsics

- *Wartenberg's sign:* 5th finger has position of abduction secondary to unopposed ulnar insertion of extensor digiti quinti
- *Duchenne's sign:* Clawing of medial two digits
- *Froment's sign:* On attempt to adduct the joint, will flex the finger
- *Tinel's sign:* Tapping over cubital canal positive for shooting pain
- *Elbow flexion test:* Flexion reproduces symptoms and symptoms regress with extension

RADIAL NERVE ENTRAPMENT (SATURDAY NIGHT PALSY)

Runs in spiral groove of humerus so is susceptible to injury after humerus fracture

- May become entrapped at radial tunnel, arcade of Frohse, or supinator channel

Symptoms: Wrist drop, decreased sensation to small region of dorsal hand

MERALGIA PARESTHETICA (LATERAL CUTANEOUS NERVE OF THIGH ENTRAPMENT)

Chronic entrapment of the lateral cutaneous nerve of thigh at the inguinal ligament, near the anterior superior iliac spine

Causes: Obesity, tight fitting belts, idiopathic

Symptoms: Sensory loss anterolateral thigh

- No motor symptoms
- Paresthesias and pain radiating down the lateral thigh to knee

Treatment: Conservative versus surgical decompression (if severe)

COMMON PERONEAL NEUROPATHY

Causes: Compression just below fibular head from prolonged lying, leg crossing, squatting, leg cast, direct compression, or mass lesions

Symptoms: Equinovarus with foot drop (plantarflexion) and inversion of the foot, paresthesias, and/or sensory loss

Signs: Foot drop/weakness on foot dorsiflexion and eversion; sensory loss on dorsum of foot.

DISTAL PERONEAL NEUROPATHY

Causes: Trauma to dorsum of foot or ankle/distal peroneal nerve, tight fitting shoe rim or strap

Symptoms: Dorsal foot paresthesias and/or sensory loss

Signs: Minimal sensory loss

TARSAL TUNNEL SYNDROME (TIBIAL NERVE ENTRAPMENT)

Causes: Fracture or dislocation of talus, calcaneus, medial malleolus, rheumatoid arthritis, tumor, diabetes

Symptoms: Aching, burning, numbness, tingling on plantar foot, distal foot, toes, and occasionally heel, paresthesias, and/or sensory loss

Signs: Positive Tinel's sign over nerve posterior to medial malleolus

- Sensory loss on plantar foot
- Atrophy of foot muscles if severe

CHAPTER 16 ■ FUNCTIONAL NEUROSURGERY AND PAIN

Nandan Lad, MD, PhD

DEEP BRAIN STIMULATION (DBS)[1]

DBS FOR PARKINSON'S DISEASE (PD)[2–10]

Nondestructive, can be performed bilaterally with low neurological morbidity (bilateral thalamotomy can precipitate cognitive decline and dysarthria), and can be modified in response to change in a patient's symptoms

■ **Parkinson's Disease (PD)**

Classic triad of resting tremor (4–8 Hz/second), cogwheel rigidity, and bradykinesia

- Due to degeneration of dopaminergic neurons of the pars compacta of the substantia nigra

■ **Patient Selection**

As many as 50% of patients on levodopa for 5 years experience fluctuations of motor function and dyskinesia. These symptoms are especially common in patients with young onset (e.g., under the age of 50) PD; they are unique to levodopa and are not produced by the other antiparkinson drugs. Most patients experience sustained improvement of motor function in the early stages of levodopa treatment. As the disease advances, however, the effect of levodopa begins to wear off approximately 4 hours after each dose.

- Motor fluctuations are alterations between "on" periods, during which the patient enjoys a good response to medication, and "off" periods during which parkinsonian symptoms are prominent
- Dyskinesia connotes abnormal involuntary movements that are usually choreic or dystonic but, when more severe, may be ballistic or myoclonic. Dyskinesia usually appears when the patient is "on"

Rationale for surgery: Two downstream effects of nigral degeneration and dopamine deficiency in PD are excessive subthalamic nucleus (STN) excitation of the internal globus pallidus (GPi) and excessive GP inhibition of the thalamus → reduced thalamocortical activity → akinesia and rigidity

- Pallidotomy (targeted ablation of the internal segment of GP [GPi]) reverses excess pallidal inhibitory effect and improves parkinsonism
- High-frequency DBS suppresses neuronal activity

- DBS has replaced pallidotomy and thalamotomy, as DBS can safely control parkinsonian symptoms by suppressing excessive GPi or STN activity without destroying brain tissue

Effectiveness: Two prospective randomized controlled trials comparing DBS with best medical therapy have shown that bilateral DBS improves motor function in selected patients with advanced typical PD and motor fluctuations. Significant improvement in the cardinal motor features of PD (tremor, rigidity, bradykinesia, and gait) in the off-medication state is generally seen at 4 years of DBS compared with baseline

- Patients can expect a > 60% reduction in their symptoms along with > 60% reduction in medication dosing

Factors predictive of benefit: Preoperative responsiveness to levodopa is the sole robust predictor of improvement after DBS of the STN. Outcome of surgery will only be as good as the best preoperative levodopa responsiveness. Those symptoms that do not respond to levodopa preoperatively will not likely improve after surgery

Duration of benefit: Improvement following DBS of the STN and GPi usually lasts at least 3 to 5 years. Although kinesia, halting speech, postural stability, freezing of gait, and cognitive decline can worsen over time, DBS can be neuroprotective and delay progression of symptoms

Surgical complications: Serious surgical complications of DBS are infrequent. Adverse surgical events (within 1 month of the procedure) include death in 0.6% and permanent neurological sequelae in 2.8%. Additional surgical complications include infection in 5.6%, hemorrhage in 3.1%, confusion/disorientation in 2.8%, and seizures in 1.1%. DBS technology is rapidly evolving, and it is likely that hardware complications will be reduced by modifications of procedure and equipment

DBS FOR ESSENTIAL TREMOR (ET)

Electrodes are implanted in the thalamic ventral intermediate (VIM) nucleus using stereotactic methods

Effectiveness: DBS of the thalamic VIM nucleus reduces contralateral limb tremor. Two prospective trials of DBS in patients with ET found that unilateral DBS produced 60 to 90% improvement of tremor

Table 16-1 Intraoperative Misplacement of DBS Electrode and Corresponding Clinical Response. Target: STN, Disease: Parkinson's

Lead Position Relative to Target	Symptom/Sign	Anatomic Location
Deep	Depression	Substantia nigra
Medial	Dysconjugate gaze (ocular deviation)	Oculomotor (III) nucleus
Anterior/lateral	Motor weakness	Internal capsule
Posterior	Tingling	

DBS FOR DYSTONIA

DBS of the GPi is the surgical treatment of choice for children and adults with disabling primary generalized or cervical dystonia who do not respond to pharmacologic therapy or chemodenervation with botulinum toxin (botox). DBS may also be effective for focal dystonia, although the evidence is less robust than it is for generalized dystonia

FUTURE INDICATIONS FOR DBS

Depression, obsessive-compulsive disorder, Tourette syndrome, epilepsy, cluster headache and pain

BACLOFEN PUMP FOR SPINAL SPASTICITY[11]

Patient selection: Children with cerebral palsy; spinal cord injury

- Patient must undergo a successful baclofen pump trial

Pathophysiology: Imbalance of excitatory (glutamatergic) and inhibitory (GABAergic) transmission in spinal motor pathways

Surgical intervention: Intrathecal baclofen administration via a refillable pump

Mechanism of action: Increasing GABAergic transmission (intrathecal baclofen)

Outcome: Decreased spasticity, contractures, pain
- May enable wheelchair use

Complications: Related to baclofen withdrawal or overmedication

PAIN[12,13]

Several neurosurgical treatments have been designed to interrupt pain pathways or stimulate modulator systems

PAIN CLASSIFICATION[14-19]

Melzack and Wall introduced gate control theory in 1965[17]
- International Society for the Study of Pain (IASP) defines pain as "an unpleasant sensory and emotional experience," and organizes pain disorders along the following five axes: region involved, systems involved, temporal characteristics, intensity, time since onset, and etiology

Nociceptive pain: Arises from tissue damage (e.g., postoperative pain) (Figure 16–1)
- Further subdivided into somatic and visceral pain

Somatic pain: Arises from damage to body tissues
- Well localized but variable in description and experience

Visceral pain: Arises from the viscera, mediated by stretch receptors; is poorly localized, deep, dull, and cramping (e.g., appendicitis, cholecystitis, pleurisy)

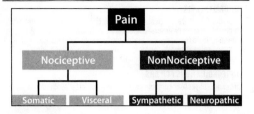

Figure 16-1 Pain

Nonnociceptive pain: Arises from abnormal neural activity secondary to disease or injury of the nervous system (Figure 16–1)

- Persists without ongoing disease (e.g., diabetic neuropathy, trigeminal neuralgia, or thalamic pain syndrome)
- Further subdivided into sympathetic and neuropathic pain

Sympathetic pain: Arises from damage to a peripheral nerve *with* autonomic change (e.g., complex regional pain syndrome I and II [reflex sympathetic dystrophy and causalgia])

Neuropathic pain: Arises from damage to a peripheral nerve *without* autonomic change (e.g., postherpetic neuralgia, neuroma formation)

- Central pain arises from abnormal central nervous system (CNS) activity (e.g., phantom limb pain, pain from spinal cord injuries, and poststroke pain)

PAIN SYNDROMES

■ Complex Regional Pain Syndrome I, II (CRPS; Reflex Sympathetic Dystrophy, Causalgia)[20]

Severe, chronic, burning pain worsening over time, exacerbated by movement, stress

- Pain out of proportion to the initial injury

Etiology:

- In Type I, initiated by *tissue injury, but no underlying nerve injury*
- Type II, *known nerve injury present;* cause for perpetuation of pain is unknown, but thought to involve the sympathetic nervous system, and possibly the immune system, and is likely multifactorial

Symptoms/Signs: Generally in one extremity

- Pain, trophic changes, vascular changes, edema, disuse (atrophy, weakness, contractures)
- Does not appear to follow any one dermatomal or nerve distribution

Stage 1: 1–3 months, severe pain, muscle spasm, hair growth, vascular alterations; *Stage 2:* 3–6 months, worsening pain, edema, nail changes, joint stiffness, decreased tone; *Stage 3:* unrelenting pain, skin/bone pain may be permanent, atrophy, contractures, limb contortion

Treatment: Sympathetic block or sympathectomy, physical therapy, psychotherapy, medications (topical analgesic, antidepressants, steroids, opioids) intrathecal opiates, spinal cord stimulation. Avoid ablative surgical procedures (e.g., dorsal root entry zone (DREZ), neurectomy, cordotomy)

CENTRAL PAIN SYNDROME

Paradoxical, unrelenting pain in the region of sensory impairment

Etiology: Stroke (e.g., VPL, VPM of the thalamus, periaqueductal gray), multiple sclerosis, tumor, seizures, trauma

Symptoms/Signs: Variability due to differences in lesion location and etiology

- Frequently burning pain, worsened by emotional stress, touch, changes in temperature
- Distal (e.g., hands/feet) may be more affected than proximal

Treatment: Neurontin, tricyclic antidepressants (e.g., nortriptyline), psychosocial counseling

■ Persistent Idiopathic (Atypical) Facial Pain[21]
Persistent aching facial pain limited to one side of the face but poorly localized, not associated with any other abnormalities

Epidemiology: 1/100K

- M = F but F more likely to seek treatment

Symptoms/Signs: Physical exam normal

Treatment: Tricyclic antidepressants, anticonvulsants (e.g., neurontin), opiates

■ Trigeminal Neuralgia (Tic Douloureux)[22]
Severe, chronic, stabbing unilateral pain, frequently triggered by skin contact, eating, talking
- No sensory loss

Epidemiology: 4/100,000

- Increased risk in multiple sclerosis

Etiology: Compression by superior cerebellar artery, anterior inferior cerebellar artery (> persistent primitive trigeminal artery > dolicoectatic basilar), demyelinating disease, tumor, idiopathic

Divisions: V2/V3 (42%), V2 (20%), V3 (17%), all (5%), V1 (2%)

DDx: Herpes zoster, dental abscess, temporal arteritis, tumor

Treatment: Antiepileptics, baclofen, gabapentin, microsurgical decompression, stereotactic radiosurgery, percutaneous rhizotomy of trigeminal/gasserian ganglion

▓ Hemifacial Spasm
Epidemiology: F > M

Etiology: Compression by anterior inferior cerebellar artery or posterior inferior cerebellar artery, tumor, idiopathic

Symptoms/Signs: Involves orbicularis oculi muscle first, then spreads to the lower facial muscles

Treatment: Microvascular decompression (MVD), botox injection

Outcome: MVD cure rate of > 80%

Complications of surgical treatment: Hearing loss, facial weakness, continued spasm, stroke, CSF leak

▓ Glossopharyngeal Neuralgia
Symptoms/Signs: Sharp, stabbing, recurrent pain in throat, tongue, and middle ear, triggered by actions such as swallowing, coughing, talking

Etiology: PICA compression of CN IX at the dorsal root entry zone, idiopathic, demyelinating disease (e.g., multiple sclerosis), tumor, Eagle's syndrome (extracranial compression by elongated styloid process)

Treatment: Anticonvulsants (e.g., gabapentin, carbamazepine), microvascular decompression, division of the glossopharyngeal and upper 1/3 of the vagus

Complications of surgical treatment: Dysphagia, dysphonia

▓ Occipital Neuralgia[23]
Piercing, electric pain in the distribution of the greater and lesser occipital nerves

Etiology: Nerve compression, trauma, tumor, inflammation, infection, diabetes, vasculitis, idiopathic

Symptoms/Signs: Scalp pain extending to behind eyes

- Allodynia, photophobia
- Pain relieved with nerve block

Treatment: Massage, rest, muscle relaxants, nerve block, steroid injection, occipital nerve stimulation, occipital neurectomy

Complications of surgical treatment: Deafferation pain (especially if bilateral), scalp numbness, infection

SURGICAL TREATMENT OF PAIN SYNDROMES[24]
▓ Cordotomy
Lesion: A lesion in the anterolateral quadrant of the spinal cord (spinothalamic tract), which carries pain signals from the contralateral body to the thalamus; a percutaneous modification makes this a minimally invasive procedure for an experienced operator

Patient selection: Generally reserved for cancer patients with limited life expectancy, unilateral somatic pain (not for deafferation), below the C5 dermatome (e.g. lumbosacral plexopathy from tumor invasion). Pain from lung cancer and mesothelioma may be amenable to high cervical cordotomy. Bilateral cordotomy may be used for bilateral or midline pain conditions, but not at high cervical levels due to the complication of Ondine's curse

Outcome: Pain relief is immediate and allows for decreased intake of opiates. Initial success with cordotomy is high (70–100%), but recurrence of pain is common months to years later (therefore, best for patients with limited life expectancy)

Complications: Corticospinal and reticulospinal tracts are also located in the anterolateral quadrant. Thus, voluntary and involuntary respiration may be affected by high cordotomy (Ondine's curse). Autonomic fiber disruption interferes with bowel and bladder function in approximately 2% of patients. Persistent paresis is also seen in 2%. These complications are more likely when bilateral lesions are made

■ Dorsal Rhizotomy

Lesion: Interruption of dorsal roots blocks all regional sensation, including pain. A highly selective rhizotomy involves small incisions in the intermediate posterolateral sulcus of the cord, adjacent to the dorsal root entry sites. Pain sensation may be selectively interrupted without loss of normal sensation or proprioception

Patient selection: Best for patients with pain from tumor invasion (e.g., chest wall). As with intrathecal neurolysis, rhizotomy is not effective for purely neuropathic pain; may consider for post herpetic neuralgia; must treat the level above and below the pain distribution

Outcome: Results in pain relief in 50–80% of patients

Complications: Motor function is impaired if proprioception is blocked. Thus, this procedure must be limited to several dermatomes serving the trunk or functionless limbs

■ Dorsal Root Entry Zone Lesioning (DREZ)

Lesion: Destruction of Lissauer's tract and outer Rexed laminae, preventing the development of deafferentation pain

Patient selection: Best for radicular pain syndromes after severe neurological injury

- Classically used to treat pain from brachial or lumbar plexus avulsion, but has also been successfully applied to phantom limb pain, radiation plexopathy, and postherpetic neuralgia
- Should have no potential for recovery of function

Outcome: Brachial plexus avulsion pain successfully treated in > 50% of cases

■ Cranial Rhizotomy

Lesion: Radiation or resection of affected nerve, e.g., percutaneous and open rhizotomies of the glossopharyngeal, trigeminal, spinal accessory nerve

Surgical section of the nerve, thermal, and chemical ablation have also been used

Patient selection: Tumor growth causing somatic or neuralgic orofacial pain, torticollis

Outcome: Prolonged pain relief, neurological deficit is expected

Complications: Recurrent pain is common

■ Commissural Myelotomy

Lesion: Crossing nociceptive fibers (spinothalamic tract) and possibly a polysynaptic pain pathway lie in the anterior commissure of the spinal cord; a small lesion of the spinal commissure at the C2 level

Patient selection: Often effective for pelvic, perineal, or bilateral leg pain in terminal patients. Similar to cordotomy, this procedure is employed to prevent midline and visceral pain below the level of the lesion from reaching the midbrain

Outcome: 70% of well-selected patients achieve relief from commissural myelotomy

Complications: Weakness, sphincter disturbances, and respiratory dysfunction less likely with this procedure than with cordotomy; pain recurs over time

■ Hypophysectomy

Lesion: Ablation of the pituitary

- Analgesic mechanism still unknown but not associated with tumor regression

Patient selection: Widespread pain due to metastatic cancer (introduced in 1953 for the treatment of breast and prostate tumors)

Outcome: Rapid onset of analgesia

■ Neurostimulation

Unlike neuroablation, neurostimulation is reversible and may be patient controlled

Mechanism of action: Possible mechanisms of stimulation-induced analgesia are numerous, including inhibitory neurotransmitter release, sensory conduction blockade, dorsal horn "gate" closure, and others

Location: Stimulation of thalamic nuclei is useful for some neuropathic pain conditions, but requires considerable expertise for lead placement. The periaqueductal and periventricular gray matter contains receptors for opioids. DBS of these regions produces naloxone-reversible analgesia

Outcome: Motor and sensory functions are generally preserved with stimulatory procedures

■ Spinal Cord Stimulation

Procedure: A set of electrodes is inserted into the epidural space to deliver electrical stimulation to the appropriate segment of the spinal cord. The electrodes are then connected to an implantable pulse generator

Location: Lower extremity radicular pain should be treated with placement of the stimulator over the spinal cord dorsal columns lumbar enlargement area (T10–11)

- Minimize stimulation of the dorsal roots

Patient selection: Anesthesiologists and neurosurgeons use spinal cord stimulation (SCS) to treat intractable, regional neuropathic pain. SCS is primarily used for treatment of pain from failed back surgery syndrome (FBSS) or complex regional pain syndrome (CRPS)

Intraventricular Opioid Delivery
Procedure: Morphine may be injected into the cerebral ventricles after placement of an Ommaya reservoir or with a continuous infusion pump

Patient selection: Appropriate for certain patients with pain from head and neck cancer, but no studies have demonstrated superiority of intraventricular over systemic opioid delivery

Outcome: 50–90% of patients obtain good to excellent initial relief

Thoracic Sympathectomy
Lesion: Thoracic sympathetic chain via thorascopy

Patient selection: Hyperhidrosis

Complications: Compensatory hyperhidrosis of other body parts

- Horner's syndrome if T1 sympathetic ganglia are involved

Intrathecal Pain Pump[25]
For treatment of pain without the systemic side effects of opioid medication

Patient selection: Generally reserved for cancer patients with limited life expectancy, but greater than 3 months

- Requires ongoing maintenance and refilling of the pump
- Can also be considered for a wide variety of nonmalignant pain
- Patients must first be tested with an external pump

Outcome: Reduction in nonmalignant pain was good or excellent (pain decrease > 50%) in 70%

Complications: Infection, technical problems (catheter or pump)

Intrathecal Baclofen Pump
For treatment of severe spasticity

Patient selection: Severe spasticity from cerebral or spinal origin, unresponsive to oral antispastic medications or for those who do not tolerate side effects

Microvascular Decompression
Indications: For treatment of hemifacial spasm, trigeminal neuralgia, glossopharyngeal neuralgia, torticollis (Table 16-2)

Table 16-2 Vascular Compression of Cranial Nerves

Clinical Syndrome	CN	Common Offending Vessel
Trigeminal Neuralgia	V	Superior Cerebellar Artery
Hemifacial Spasm	VII	Anterior Inferior Cerebellar Artery
Glossopharyngeal Neuralgia	XII	Posterior Inferior Cerebellar Artery

Etiology: Compression of dorsal root entry zone by vessel (must first rule out mass lesion or multiple sclerosis)

Approach: Retrosigmoid

- May consider opening the cisterna magna for improved CSF drainage

Complications: Hearing loss (coagulation of the labyrinthine artery, branch of the AICA), facial paresis/plegia, CSF leak, facial sensory deficit, hemorrhage, infarct

■ Motor Cortex Stimulation
Transdural electrical stimulation of the precentral gyrus thought to mediate pain through retrograde thalamic stimulation pathways
- Patients must undergo a successful trial prior to permanent implantation
- Risks: Infection, hematoma, painful stimulation, ineffective pain relief, CSF leak

CHAPTER 17 ■ NEUROSURGICAL APPROACHES

Lewis Hou, MD

FRONTOTEMPORAL

Includes pterional and variants; see Figure 17-1

Indications
- Tumor: Tumors in the lateral frontal lobe, temporal lobe, or suprasellar regions
- Vascular: Aneurysms (Acom, Pcom, ICA, MCA, anterior choroidal, ophthalmic, some basilar tip)
- Others: Anterior temporal lobectomy

Position: Supine

- Ipsilateral shoulder roll
- Head turned away 15–45°
- Head vertex declination and extension to keep malar eminence the highest point

Incision: Curved incision from root of zygoma (1 cm or less anterior to the ear) to widow's peak

- Care is made to stay posterior to hair line when possible
- Extent of incision depends on location of pathology and exposure needed

Craniotomy: Burr holes in the anatomic keyhole, low temporal squamosal region, and posterior frontal (optional)

- Size of craniotomy varies depending on the location of the pathology and exposure needed
- Removal of sphenoid ridge and occasionally the anterior clinoid process may be needed for adequate exposure of internal carotid artery for proximal control during clipping of anterior circulation aneurysms

■ Pearls

1. Lumbar drain placement for clipping of ruptured aneurysm minimizes need for retraction and unexpected brain swelling
2. Extending the head with its vertex down to keep the malar eminence at the apex is crucial to allow access to the base of the skull without significant retraction of the frontal lobe
3. During clipping of ruptured PCom aneurysms, place temporal lobe retractor last to decrease the risk of sudden intraoperative rupturing before securing proximal control

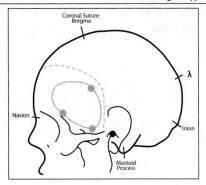

Figure 17-1 Frontotemporal Approach

▨ Caution

1. Preoperative review of imaging studies to identify and avoid breaching of the frontal sinus
2. Avoid excessive head turning by using appropriate shoulder roll to minimize kinking of the internal jugular veins, thereby compromising venous return
3. Caution should be taken to avoid entering into the orbit during burr hole placement or drilling of the sphenoid ridge
4. Avoid injury of the frontal branch of the facial nerve by preserving fat pad

SUBFRONTAL (Figure 17-2)

Indications

- Tumor: Meningioma (olfactory groove, tuberculum sellar), craniopharyngioma, nasopharyngeal carcinoma
- Vascular: Rare
- Others: Traumatic CSF leak repair

Positioning: Supine

- Head extended
- Flex head of bed to keep head above heart level

Incision: Bicoronal incision

Craniotomy: Burr holes placed in bilateral anatomic key holes and over anterior superior sagittal sinus

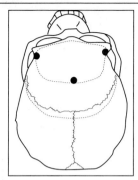

Figure 17-2 Subfrontal Approach

■ **Pearls**
1. Placement of lumbar drain or frontal ventriculostomy drain (Kocher's point) in addition to hyperosmolar diuresis can drastically minimize need for frontal lobe retraction
2. Preservation and preparation of pericranial flap provides additional option for prevention of CSF leak
3. Cranialization of frontal sinuses often necessary

■ **Caution**
1. Minimize frontal lobe retraction
2. Prepare to encounter superior sagittal sinus bleed when opening dura
3. Avoid iatrogenic injury to anterior cerebral arteries and optic apparatus
4. Postoperative CSF leak

INTERHEMISPHERIC (Figure 17-3)

Indications

- Tumor: Metastastic tumors, intraventricular tumors (central neurocytoma, colloid cyst, meningioma)
- Vascular: Pericallosal aneruysms, cavernous malformations, arteriovenous malformations
- Others: Corpus callosotomy, placement of interhemispheric epileptic monitoring grids

Position: Patient is placed in supine position

- Head kept straight in neutral position
- Head of bed flexed to give optimal angle according to location of the lesion

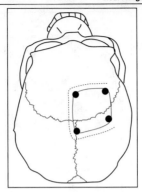

Figure 17-3 Interhemispheric Approach

Incision: Horseshoe (inverted U shape) incision, with base toward ipsilateral side

Craniotomy: Burr holes over superior sagittal sinus and lateral frontal/parietal bone (See Figure 17-3). Longitudinal position (anterior/posterior) of the craniotomy depends on the location of the pathology. In general, the craniotomy is placed 2/3 anterior and 1/3 posterior over the coronal suture as illustrated

■ Pearls

1. Image-guided navigation can be helpful in localization of lesion of interest; allows early identification of superior sagittal sinus
2. During craniotomy portion, perform cut over superior sagittal sinus last
3. Base durotomy toward the superior sagittal sinus
4. Identification of four anterior cerebral artery branches helps to localize the corpus callosum
5. Familiarity of the intraventricular anatomy is crucial in helping to determine if the correct (ipsilateral rather than contralateral) ventricle has been entered

■ Caution

1. Minimize sacrificing any venous drainage to the superior sagittal sinus
2. Dural opening can often be complicated by draining veins or by presence of arachnoid granulation
3. Avoid iatrogenic injury to the anterior cerebral arteries

TEMPORAL/SUBTEMPORAL (Figure 17-4)

Indications

- Tumor: Tumors in the medial, posterior, or inferior temporal lobe
- Vascular: Basilar tip (at or below posterior clinoid) and upper 3rd basilar trunk, proximal PCA/SCA aneurysms, lateral midbrain cavernous malformations
- Others: Pathologies near the tentorial notch

Position: Patient placed supine, with a roll placed under the ipsilateral shoulder

- Head turned to keep parallel to the floor
- Slight lateral flexion is performed toward the floor to allow temporal lobe to fall away from floor of middle fossa

Incision: Inverted U-shaped incision based at the ear or linear vertical incision starting just anterior to the ear

- Care is taken to avoid injury to the frontal branch of the facial nerve during the former incision by staying above the zygoma

Craniotomy: Burr holes are placed just above the floor of middle fossa

- After bone flap is removed, a rangeur is used to remove the remainder of the temporal squamous bone until the middle fossa floor is encountered

▓ Pearls

1. Placement of lumbar drain and early initiation of hyperosmolar diuresis are crucial in order to minimize need for retraction of the temporal lobe
2. Compulsive waxing of exposed air cells may reduce the risk of postoperative CSF leak

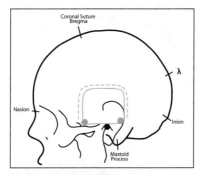

Figure 17-4 Temporal/Subtemporal Approach

■ **Caution**

1. Injury to the frontal branch of facial nerve during incision as described
2. Avoid transecting the trochlear nerve during manipulation of the tentorium
3. Caution should be taken to avoid injury to the vein of Labbé

LATERAL SUBOCCIPITAL INCLUDING RETROMASTOID AND RETROSIGMOID

See Figure 17-5

Indications

- Tumor: Cerebellopontine angle tumors including schwannomas (vestibular, trigeminal, facial), meningiomas and epidermoids
- Cerebellar lesions such as metastasis, cerebellar astrocytomas, and hemangioblastomas
- Vascular: Vertebrobasilar junction and PICA aneurysms, pontine cavernous malformations
- Others: Microvascular decompression for trigeminal neuralgia, glossopharyngeal neuralgia, and hemifacial spasm

Position: Supine with large shoulder roll or lateral decubitus position

- Head turned contralaterally and kept parallel to the floor
- Ipsilateral shoulder taped caudally to maximize room for the surgeon

Incision: Linear vertical incision approximately two finger breadths posterior to the ear, extending from level of the top of the ear to level of the mastoid tip

- For vertebral basilar aneurysms or ventral clival tumors, a reverse hockey stick or S-shaped incision is made

Craniotomy: Single burr hole just inferior and posterior the asterion is made

- Intersection between sigmoid and tranverse sinuses is identified
- Craniotomy or craniectomy flap is made posteroinferiorly
- Depending on the lesion location, the craniotomy may or may not need to extend to the foramen magnum
- For vertebrobasilar or PICA aneurysms, C1 hemilaminectomy may be necessary

■ **Pearls**

1. Careful positioning of the patient is crucial in optimizing intraoperative exposure
2. Hyperosmolar diuresis is sometimes required to achieve brain relaxation
3. Significant relaxation can be achieved with CSF drainage from the cisterna magnum
4. Petrosal veins can be sacrificed to improve exposure with minimal neurologic sequela

■ **Caution**

1. Avoid excessive head turning by using appropriate shoulder roll to minimize kinking of the internal jugular veins, thereby compromising venous return
2. Care should be taken to avoid tension on the facial nerve during cerebellar retraction

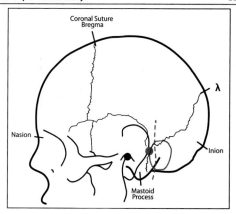

Figure 17-5 Lateral Suboccipital Including Retromastoid and Retrosigmoid

SUBOCCIPITAL CRANIOTOMOY (Figure 17-6)

Indications

- Tumors: Cerebellar region tumors (astrocytoma, hemangioblastoma, metastasis, ependymoma, medulloblastoma), pineal region tumors, tentorial/falcine meningioma
- Vascular: Distal PICA-PICA anastamosis; occipital and cerebellar AVM/ cavernous malformation
- Others: Chiari malformation decompression, cerebellar hematoma evacuation

Position: Patient placed in prone position with appropriate bolsters and padding

- Head flexed and the neck placed in the military position
- Minimum two finger breadths should be maintained between the chin and the chest

Incision: Midline vertical incision extending from the inion to C2

Craniotomy: Two burr holes are placed just below the transverse sinuses

- Craniotomy flap made by passing the craniotome first inferolaterally then inferomedially toward the foramen magnum
- For Chiari decompression, the burr holes are made half way between the inion and the Foramen Magnum

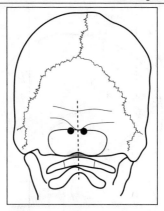

Figure 17-6 Occipital/Suboccipital Approach

■ **Pearl**
1. Meticulous dural closure and multilayer muscle closure can minimize development of postoperative pseudomeningocele
2. Close postoperative monitoring for hydrocephalus and hemorrhage is crucial in patients with posterior fossa procedures

■ **Caution**
1. Avoid excessive flexion of the neck, which can compromise venous return
2. Raising the head of the table above the heart improves venous return, which can help minimize intraoperative bleeding
3. Care should be taken to avoid injury to vertebral arteries during initial dissection and C1 laminectomy

CHAPTER 18 ■ NEUROSURGICAL DICTATION TEMPLATES

Robert Lober, MD, PhD

Melanie G. Hayden Gephart, MD, MAS

GENERAL DICTATION FORMAT

1. Your name and ID #
2. Patient's name and ID #
3. Date of service
4. Preoperative diagnosis
5. Postoperative diagnosis
6. Primary surgeon(s)
7. Assistants
8. Indication for procedure
9. Operation performed (CPT code)
10. Procedure in detail
11. Anesthesia (Include name of anesthesiologist)
12. Intraoperative findings
13. Fluids
14. Estimated blood loss
15. Urine output
16. Drains/tubes (type and site)
17. Specimens/cultures
18. Complications
19. Disposition
20. Presence of attending surgeon

COMMON SECTIONS

■ Indications for Procedure

(Pt Name) is a (age) year old (gender) with (comorbidities) who presented to (hospital/clinic/ER) with (signs/symptoms). (Provide further detail on clinical course to date). (Diagnostic study) showed (findings). (Explain why the surgery is indicated to treat patient). All risks, benefits, and alternatives of this procedure were discussed in detail with the (patient/responsible party). Risks discussed included but were not limited to (list). Understanding these risks and expected outcomes, the (patient/responsible party) elected to proceed. Informed consent paperwork was signed and properly filed

■ Procedure in Detail

First step: After confirming patient identification and informed consent by the (patient/responsible party), the patient was premedicated, taken to the operating room, and placed in the (supine/prone/lateral) position on the operating table. Prior to incision, the patient was again positively identified and a full "time out" was undertaken with the attending physician present, which included a review of the patient's name, medical record number, date of birth, operative side and site, correct patient films, SCD prophylaxis and perioperative antibiotics. (General endotracheal/monitored/LMA) anesthesia was established, and appropriate lines and monitors were placed. Eyes were taped shut following placement of ointment to prevent corneal abrasion. Antibiotic prophylaxis with (ceftriaxone/Kefzol/vancomycin) was given 30 min prior to incision. All bony prominences and peripheral nerves were appropriately padded and the patient was covered (with a Bair hugger) to maintain body warmth. Foley catheter was placed. (Patient positioning). (Placement of neuromonitoring electrodes). Hair was clipped over the area of the planned incision. A pre-prep was performed with (alcohol), imaging and laterality were confirmed, and the planned incision was drawn. Patient was prepped and draped in the standard sterile fashion. (Xcc) of local anesthetic (X% lidocaine and epinephrine at 1:X) was infiltrated along the line of the drawn skin incision. The incision was opened sharply with a (10) blade and hemostasis was achieved utilizing monopolar and bipolar electrocautery

Sterotaxis (CPT 61795, 01169T): Stereotactic (MRI/CT) performed prior to surgery was loaded onto the (Company) neuro-navigation system. The reference frame for the stereotactic navigation device was attached to the base-mount of the Mayfield and the fiducial points were registered in the three-dimensional coordinate system of the computer navigational system. Utilizing the previously obtained images and the (feducials/anatomic landmarks), 3-D images were reconstructed. The final accuracy of the registration was (< X cm). Prior to incision, vital structures and anatomic landmarks, in relation to the target lesion were outlined. An incision and trajectory were planned following the stereotactic guide. The neuronavigational probe was utilized throughout the duration of the case to ensure appropriate targeting and trajectory

Neuromonitoring (CPT 95925 SSEP–UE), 95926 (SSEP–LE), 95928 (Motor Evoked–UE), 95929 (Motor Evoked–LE): Intraoperative monitoring was then initiated with (company, size) grid placed over the (anatomical location). Areas of (motor cortex, language) were mapped out utilizing the (Ojemann) stimulator. The neuromonitoring team headed by Dr. (neurologist) assisted in intraoperative electrocorticography. During the case and upon final closure there was (no change in MEP/SSEP)

Tumor resection (varies greatly) CPT 61605-8, 69990 (microsurgery): The (Greenberg) retractor was fixed to the Mayfield. Maleable retractors with corresponding hemostatic material (company) were prepared. The dura was opened in a (C-shaped/stellar) manner. Following opening of the dura, the suctions were changed to fenestrated (5/7-) French. The brain and dura were kept moist with frequent irrigation of saline. The arachnoid and pia of the cortex at the confirmed entry site was coagulated with bipolar electro-cautery. The operative microscope was essential for resection of the tumor and preservation of normal anatomy. It was draped in a sterile manner and brought into the operative field. A corticectomy was performed and dis-section was taken down to the level of the (lesion). (Describe findings). An uncauterized section of the mass was resected with a (micropituitary) and sent to neuropathology for frozen diagnosis. The bipolar electrocau-tery and microscissors were utilized to identify a plane around the lesion. A CUSA (cored out/collapsed) the lesion. Neuronavigation throughout the case ensured protection of crucial structures, and excision of the lesion to the extent determined to be safe. All visualized major vessels were well preserved

Cranial Closure - CPT 20926: Meticulous hemostasis was obtained with bipo-lar and monopolar electrocautery, as well as gelatin hemostatic matrix and foam. The dura was carefully (reapproximated/water-tight closure) with 4-0 Neurolon. (Synthetic dural graft/periostioum was utilized to close the dura Tissue graft)Synthetic dural matrix (company) and hydrogel dural sealant (company) were applied to the closed dura. (Tack-up sutures were placed in the dura with 4-0 Neurolon, and passed through newly drilled holes in the bone flap). The bone flap was fitted with (#) (company) titanium plates and (#) screws and secured back to the patient's skull. The wound was copiously irri-gated with antibiotic irrigation. After again confirming hemostasis, the galea was closed with inverted interrupted stitches utilizing (X)-0 (Vicryl) suture. The skin was approximated with (staples/sutures). (Drains were sutured in place with (X-0 nylon suture). A sterile dressing was placed over the closed incision and the dressings were removed.

Spine closure: Meticulous hemostasis was obtained with bipolar and monop-olar electrocautery, as well as gelatin hemostatic matrix and foam. [The dura was closed in a watertight manner with (6-0 Gortex). Hydrogel dural sealant (company) was applied to the closed dura]. The wound was care-fully but copiously irrigated with antibiotic irrigation. (A [Jackson-Pratt/7" hemovac] drain was placed in the (subfacial/facial/subcutaneous) space). After again confirming hemostasis, the wound was closed in a multiple lay-ers including muscle (0 Vicryl), fascia (0 Vicryl), subcutaneous tissue (2-0 Vicryl). The skin was closed with (inverted interrupted stitches utilizing 3-0 Vicryl suture/staples/sutures). (Drains were sutured in pace with (X-0 nylon suture). A sterile dressing was placed over the closed incision and the drapes were removed

Final step: All needle, sponge, and instrument counts were correct times two prior to the final closure of the incision. The patient tolerated the procedure well and there were no intraoperative complications. He was (extubated) and taken to the (PACU/ICU) in (stable/ guarded) condition

I. CSF DIVERSION

A. VENTRICULOPERITONEAL SHUNT (CPT 62223): OCCIPITAL APPROACH

1. The patient was positioned supine with the head (placed on a gel horse-shoe headrest and) turned to the (left). The (right) occipital area of the head was shaved. A marker was placed at the glabella. A roll was placed beneath the shoulders to elevate the chest, creating a straight trajectory for subcutaneous passage of the abdominal catheter. Incisions were drawn at the entry point for the ventricular catheter (U-shaped), and at the abdomen in the upper (right) quadrant at the edge of the rectus sheath. The (right) occipital area and ipsilateral neck, chest, and abdomen were then prepped and draped in the usual manner.

2. All parts of the shunt system were primed with antibiotic irrigation, and kept submerged in antibiotic irrigation, covered in a blue towel on the back table until requested. Traffic in and out of the OR was restricted. Handling of the shunt components was kept to an absolute minimum.

3. (X cc) of local anesthetic (X% lidocaine and epinephrine at 1:X) was infiltrated along the line of the drawn abdominal incision. The incision was opened sharply with a (15) blade and hemostasis was achieved utilizing monopolar and bipolar electrocautery. Using (Metzenbaum), the incision was taken down through the subcutaneous tissue to the anterior rectus sheath. At the edge of the rectus abdominus, the anterior rectus sheath was incised, and the muscle was divided with a muscle-splitting dissection using hemostats. The posterior rectus sheath was identified and held with two snaps. A purse string stitch of (suture type) was placed around two snaps and the posterior rectus sheath and peritoneum were incised with a clean (15) blade. A red rubber catheter was introduced intraperitoneally without resistance. When filled with saline, the red rubber catheter drained immediately. The abdomen was covered with blue towels. Gloves were cleaned with antibiotic soaked sponge.

4. After subcutaneous infiltration with (X cc) of local anesthetic (X% lidocaine and epinephrine at 1:X), a curvilinear skin incision was made at the (right) occiput. The incision was opened sharply with a (15) blade and hemostasis was achieved utilizing monopolar and bipolar electrocautery. The underlying periosteum was preserved. A (4-0 Neurolon) stitch retracted skin and galea and was snapped to the drape. A caudal subcutaneous pocket was made with the Metzenbaum scissors, and the cervical fascia inferior to this pocket was penetrated. The pericranium was incised with monocautery and a (X cm) burr hole was created with a (perforator/ M8). Bone wax was applied and the underlying dura was coagulated.

5. A tunneling device created a subcutaneous tract from the (right) occipital incision, over the clavicle, down to the abdominal incision. A heavy (0) suture was tied to the tunneling device and drawn up through the tract. The peritoneal catheter was tied to the heavy suture and then brought down from the cranial incision with antibiotic irrigation into the tract. The distal catheter was placed in an antibiotic soaked sponge and covered with a blue towel.

6. The (company, setting) valve tip was inserted into the proximal portion of the abdominal catheter and secured with a (2-0 silk) stitch. The valve was positioned in the subcutaneous pocket.

7. Attention was then directed to the ventricular portion of the shunt. The previously cauterized dura was carefully opened with an (11) blade. (Manually guided by the glabellar marker/using sterotactic guidance), the occipital horn of the lateral ventricle was entered with an Elsberg cannula, which retrieved clear CSF. This was collected for glucose, protein, cell count, Gram stain, and cultures. Care was taken not to overdrain the ventricle.

8. (A [X]-mm [company] endoscope within the ventricular catheter was inserted to confirm intraventricular location. The catheter was positioned at the (junction of the foramen of Monro and the 3rd ventricle/anterior horn of the lateral ventricle). The endoscope was removed and the ventricular catheter was trimmed to (X cm). The ventricular catheter was connected to the valve and secured with a (2-0 silk) suture. This area was then anchored to the pericranium with a 3-0 silk stitch.

9. Flow from the ventricle to the distal tubing was confirmed. The abdominal catheter was then introduced intraperitoneally and secured with the a purse string suture placed in the peritoneum and posterior rectus sheath. The anterior rectus sheath was closed with (a running 3-0 Vicryl) stitch.

10. Both incisions were copiously irrigated with warm saline with bacitracin, and then closed with interrupted inverted (4-0 Vicryl) in the subcutaneous layer and running (4-0 nylon) suture in the skin. Sterile dressings were applied and the drapes were removed.

B. ENDOSCOPIC THIRD VENTRICULOSTOMY (CPT 62200)

1. The patient was positioned supine with the head in neutral position, slightly extended, and in (Mayfield) pins. The right frontal area overlying the coronal suture in the midpupillary line was then shaved. A marker was placed at the glabella. The area was prepped and draped in the usual manner. A Mayo stand was brought over the face to protect the airway. A linear incision extending along the midpupillary line, over the (right) coronal suture, was drawn with a marking pen.

2. (X cc) of local anesthetic (X% lidocaine and epinephrine at 1:X) was infiltrated along the line of the drawn incision. The incision was opened sharply with a (15) blade and hemostasis was achieved utilizing monopolar and bipolar electrocautery. A self-retracting Wheatlander retractor was placed. A (X cm) burr hole was created with a (perforator/M8). Bone wax was applied and the underlying dura was coagulated.

3. The previously coagulated dura was carefully opened with an (11) blade. The pia was also coagulated and opened with an (11) blade.

4. (Manually guided by the glabellar marker/using sterotactic guidance), the (right) frontal horn of the lateral ventricle was cannulated with a 14-gauge peel-away catheter. This retrieved clear CSF under (moderate/high) pressure. This was collected for glucose, protein, cell count, Gram stain, and

cultures. Care was taken not to overdrain the ventricle. The stylet was then removed and replaced with an endoscope.

5. We proceeded to endoscopically identify the foramen of Monro, choroid plexus, mammillary bodies, infundibular recess, and ependyma overlying the floor of the 3rd ventricle.

6. A region of avascular ependyma anterior to the mammillary bodies, on the floor of the 3rd ventricle was fenestrated with a guide wire. The hole was dilated with a (Cook catheter/Fogarty balloon). The floor became markedly pulsatile, consistent with a gradient of CSF flow. Upon advancing the endoscope through the floor of the 3rd ventricle, the posterior clinoid, prepontine cistern, clivus, and basilar artery could be seen below the fenestration, (with/without) significant arachnoidal adhesions.

7. The endoscope and peel-away catheter were removed, watching closely on exiting for any potential hemorrhage. The cortical opening and burr hole were sealed with hemostatic absorbable gelatin foam.

8. The incision was irrigated thoroughly with warm saline/antibiotic solution, and then closed with interrupted inverted (4-0 Vicryl) in the subcutaneous layer and running (4-0 nylon) suture in the skin. Sterile dressings were applied and the drapes were removed.

C. OMMAYA RESERVOIR PLACEMENT (CPT 61215)

1. The patient was positioned supine with the head in neutral position, slightly extended, and in (Mayfield head clamp/Horseshoe head rest). The right frontal area overlying the coronal suture in the midpupillary line was then shaved. A marker was placed at the glabella. The area was prepped and draped in the usual manner. A Mayo stand was brought over the face to protect the airway. A linear incision extending along the midpupillary line, over the (right) coronal suture, was drawn with a marking pen.

2. (X cc) of local anesthetic (X% lidocaine and epinephrine at 1:X) was infiltrated along the line of the drawn incision. The incision was opened sharply with a (10) blade and hemostasis was achieved utilizing monopolar and bipolar electrocautery. A self-retracting Wheatlander retractor was placed. A (X cm) burr hole was created with a (perforator/M8). Bone wax was applied and the underlying dura was coagulated.

3. The previously coagulated dura was carefully opened with an (11) blade. The pia was then also coagulated and opened with an (11) blade.

4. (Manually guided by the glabellar marker/using sterotactic guidance), the (right) frontal horn of the lateral ventricle was cannulated with the ventricular catheter. This retrieved clear CSF under (moderate/high) pressure. This was collected for glucose, protein, cell count, Gram stain, and cultures. Care was taken not to overdrain the ventricle. Utilizing (sterotactic guidance/anatomical landmarks), the ventricular catheter was inserted to (X cm).

5. The ventricular catheter was securely attached to the Ommaya reservoir with a (2-0 silk) suture. The reservoir was tested with a (X)-gauge butterfly needle and CSF was readily obtained. The cortical opening and burr hole were sealed with hemostatic absorbable gelatin foam.

6. The incision was irrigated thoroughly with warm saline/antibiotic solution, and then closed with interrupted inverted (4-0 Vicryl) in the subcutaneous layer and running (4-0 nylon) suture in the skin. Sterile dressings were applied and the drapes were removed.

II. CRANIOTOMY

A. EMERGENT CRANIOTOMY/ECTOMY FOR ACUTE SUBDURAL OR EPIDURAL HEMATOMA EVACUATION (CPT 61312), DECOMPRESSIVE HEMICRANIECTOMY (CPT 61322)

1. Increased intracranial pressure was treated with moderate hyperventilation and mannitol 0.5–1 gm/kg.
2. The patient was placed supine and the head was turned to the (left) and placed in Mayfield three-point fixation with 10–15° of elevation and a roll beneath the (right) shoulder. The neck position was checked to ensure no compression of the jugular veins. The (right) side of the head was generously shaved, then prepped and draped in the usual sterile fashion.
3. (X cc) of local anesthetic (X% lidocaine and epinephrine at 1:X) was infiltrated along the line of the drawn incision. An incision was made beginning 1 cm anterior to the right tragus and at the root of the zygoma, curving posteriorly above the helix of the ear around the posterior temporal area, to the frontal midline in a reverse "question mark." Hemostasis was achieved with (electrocautery).
4. Using a periosteal elevator and electrocautery, the scalp flap was elevated with the temporalis muscle, retracted, and secured with (towel clips/fish hooks and rubber bands).
5. An initial burr hole was made in the temporal squamosa with a (perforator/X mm round burr) drill. Bone wax was applied for hemostasis. Three additional burr holes were made. A Penfield #3 was utilized to free the dura from the bone edge. A fronto-temporal-parietal craniotomy with its superior edge 1 cm lateral to midline was then completed with a (craniotome) drill bit. The bone flap was elevated while stripping dura with a Penfield #. 3 (and removed for sterile cryopreservation/storage in the abdomen).
6. The dura was irrigated to remove bone dust and hemostasis was achieved with bipolar electrocautery. Holes were drilled in the outer table of the craniotomy margins, through which 4-0 silk dural tenting sutures were placed circumferentially. Strips of absorbable hemostatic matrix were placed at the edges of exposed dura.
7. The dura was elevated with a sharp hook, and opened with a #11 blade. A (stellate/C-shaped) incision was extended with Metzenbaum scissors and dural forceps. Any hemorrhage of the underlying brain parenchyma or vasculature was cauterized.
8. An artificial dural graft was placed on the brain.
9. The bone flap was replaced and secured with titanium plates and screws
10. Crani closure.

B. BURR HOLES FOR DRAINAGE OF CHRONIC SUBDURAL HEMATOMA (CPT 61154)

1. The patient was placed supine and the head was turned to the (left) and placed in (Mayfield three-point fixation/Horseshoe head rest) with 10–15° of elevation and a roll beneath the (right) shoulder. The neck position was checked to ensure no compression of the jugular veins. The (right) side of the head was generously shaved. Two incisions, one anterior and one posterior were marked, keeping in mind a potential need to extend the craniotomy should significant hemorrhage be encountered. The patient was then prepped and draped in the usual sterile fashion.

2. (X cc) of local anesthetic (X% lidocaine and epinephrine at 1:X) was infiltrated along the line of the drawn incision. The incision was opened sharply with a (10) blade and hemostasis was achieved utilizing monopolar and bipolar electrocautery. A self-retracting Wheatlander retractor was placed. A (X cm) burr hole was created with a (perforator/M8). Bone wax was applied and the underlying dura was coagulated.

3. The previously coagulated dura was carefully opened in a cruciate manner with an (11) blade.

4. Dark fluid under pressure was obtained, and careful subdural irrigation ensued. Meticulate hemostasis was obtained.

5. A (Jackson-Pratt flat) drain was placed (subdural/subcutaneous) and tunneled laterally. The drain was secured to the skin.

6. Hemostasis was achieved with bipolar electrocautery.

7. Crani closure.

C. CRANIOPLASTY (CPT 62140 < 5CM, 62141 > 5CM)

1. The patient was placed supine and the head was turned to the (left) and placed in (Horseshoe head rest) with 10–15° of elevation and a roll beneath the (right) shoulder. The neck position was checked to ensure no compression of the jugular veins. The (right) side of the head was generously shaved, then prepped and draped in the usual sterile fashion.

2. (X cc) of local anesthetic (X% lidocaine and epinephrine at 1:X) was infiltrated along the line of the drawn incision. The incision was made following the old incision: beginning 1 cm anterior to the right tragus and at the root of the zygoma, curving posteriorly above the helix of the ear around the posterior temporal area, to the frontal midline in a reverse "question mark." The incision was opened sharply with a (10) blade and hemostasis was achieved utilizing monopolar and bipolar electrocautery.

3. Using a (periosteal elevator/#1 Penfield) and electrocautery, the scalp flap and periostium were elevated circumferentially from the edge of the skull defect. Substantial scarring was encountered, however, the retracted temporalis muscle was identified and separated from the dura.

4. The (bone/synthetic graft) was repositioned and ensured to fit well. It was secured with titanium plates and screws. Any prominent areas were drilled down with the (electric) drill.

5. Crani closure.

D. ORBITOZYGOMATIC APPROACH (CPT 61592)

1. The patient was placed supine and the head was turned to the (left) and placed in Mayfield three-point fixation with 10–15° of elevation and a roll beneath the (right) shoulder. The neck position was checked to ensure no compression of the jugular veins. The (right) side of the head was generously shaved, and an incision was made from 1 cm anterior to the right tragus at the inferior border of the zygoma, curving gently to a point just lateral to the midline on the left side. The patient was then prepped and draped in the usual sterile fashion.

2. (X cc) of local anesthetic (X% lidocaine and epinephrine at 1:X) was infiltrated along the line of the drawn incision. An incision was made with a (10) blade and (monopolar/bipolar) electrocautery. The scalp flap was reflected and the dissection was carried along the temporalis fascial plane to the subgaleal fat pad. The superficial fascial layer of the temporalis was incised leaving a cuff of tissue, and sharply dissected off of the skull with a Penfield #1 from inferior to superior in order to prevent muscle atrophy and minimize bleeding. This was then reflected anteriorly with the fat pad to protect the frontalis branch of the facial nerve. The periosteum of the lateral orbit and zygoma was dissected from the bone with a periosteal elevator. The periorbita was then dissected from the superolateral rim of the orbit to the level of the malar eminence. The dissection was continued medially to the supraorbital nerve, which was preserved in its (notch/foramen). The temporalis was further incised and reflected anteroinferiorly, exposing the squamosa.

3. Burr holes were made first in the temporal squamosa at the pterion (keyhole), then at the superior medial frontal bone, and finally at the posterior temporal bone with a (perforator/M8). Dura was stripped from the bone with a Penfield #3 at each burr hole. A bone flap encompassing the temporalis myofascial flap was completed with a (craniotome), and then elevated while stripping dura with a Penfield #3.

4. The intact dura was irrigated and hemostasis achieved with bipolar electrocautery. Holes were drilled in the outer table of the craniotomy margins, through which 4-0 silk circumferential dural tenting sutures were placed. Strips of absorbable hemostatic matrix were placed at the edges of exposed dura.

5. The root of the zygomatic process was obliquely cut with a cutting burr/reciprocating saw. A cut was brought anteriorly along the posterolateral rim of the malar eminence halfway to the orbit. Another cut was extended from the inferior orbital fissure to meet this. The dura was elevated to expose the superior and lateral orbit. Beginning 2 mm lateral to the supraorbital canal, the orbital roof was divided toward the superior orbital fissure. Another cut was extended from the tip of the inferior orbital fissure to the edge of the pterional craniotomy, and still another was made from the superior orbital fissure to meet this one. The orbitozygomatic flap was then elevated. The periorbita was protected with (maleable) retractors during this portion of the craniotomy. The greater wing of the sphenoid was further drilled with a (diamond) drill bit, while carefully protecting the dura.

6. The (Greenberg) retractor was fixed to the Mayfield. Maleable retractors with corresponding hemostatic material (Company) were prepared. The dura was elevated with a (sharp hook), and opened with an (#11) blade. The incision was extended with Metzenbaum scissors and dural forceps, utilizing a moist half-by-half patty to protect the underlying cortex.

7. (The operative microscope was essential for resection of the tumor and preservation of normal anatomy. It was draped in a sterile manner and brought into the operative field). The Sylvian fissure was opened via microdissection. (Further resection of the sphenoid ridge and anterior clinoid were required). (Describe identification of anatomic structures, e.g. carotid artery, cranial nerves).

8. Procedure varies; e.g., tumor resection or aneurysm clipping.

9. Crani closure.

E. PTERIONAL APPROACH (CPT 61500 SERIES, 61605-8)

1. The patient was placed supine and the head was turned to the (left) and placed in Mayfield three-point fixation with 10–15° of elevation and a roll beneath the (right) shoulder. The neck position was checked to ensure no compression of the jugular veins. The (right) side of the head was generously shaved, and an incision was made from 1 cm anterior to the right tragus at 1 cm above the zygoma, curving gently to a point just lateral to the midline on the left side. The patient was then prepped and draped in the usual sterile fashion.

2. (X cc) of local anesthetic (X% lidocaine and epinephrine at 1:X) was infiltrated along the line of the drawn incision. An incision was made with a (10) blade and (monopolar/bipolar) electrocautery. The scalp flap was reflected and the dissection was carried along the temporalis fascial plane to the subgaleal fat pad. The superficial fascial layer of the temporalis was incised leaving a cuff of tissue, and sharply dissected off of the skull with a Penfield #1 from inferior to superior in order to prevent muscle atrophy and minimize bleeding. This was then reflected anteriorly with the fat pad to protect the frontalis branch of the facial nerve. This exposed the keyhole, the root of the zygomatic arch, and the supraorbital notch. It was secured with fish hooks and rubber bands.

3. Burr holes were made in the temporal squamosa and keyhole. Dura was stripped from the bone with a Penfield #3 at each burr hole. A bone flap encompassing the temporalis myofascial flap was completed with a (craniotome), and then elevated while stripping dura with a Penfield #3. The remaining temporal squamosa was removed with Leksell rongeurs. The remaining inner table of the frontal fossa was removed with a Kerrison punch. The sphenoid wing was flattened with a (diamond) drill until the floor of the frontal and middle fossae were flush with the superior orbital fissure.

4. The intact dura was irrigated and hemostasis achieved with bipolar electrocautery. Holes were drilled in the outer table of the craniotomy margins, through which (4-0 Neurolon) circumferential dural tenting sutures were placed. Strips of absorbable hemostatic matrix were placed at the edges of exposed dura.

5. The (Greenberg) retractor was fixed to the mayfield. Maleable retractors with corresponding hemostatic material (company) were prepared. The dura was elevated with a (sharp hook), and opened with an (#11) blade. The incision was extended with Metzenbaum scissors and dural forceps, utilizing a moist half-by-half patty to protect the underlying cortex.
6. (The operative microscope was essential for resection of the tumor and preservation of normal anatomy. It was draped in a sterile manner and brought into the operative field). The Sylvian fissure was opened via microdissection. (Further resection of the sphenoid ridge and anterior clinoid were required). (Describe identification of anatomic structues, e.g. carotid artery, cranial nerves).
7. Procedure varies; e.g., tumor resection or aneurysm clipping
8. Crani closure.

F. INTERHEMISPHERIC TRANSCALLOSAL APPROACH (CPT 61500 SERIES)

**Measurements vary depending upon the location of the intracranial pathology

1. The patient was placed supine in the lounge chair position with the head elevated in three-point fixation. The head was shaved, and a skin incision was drawn starting at a point 1.5 cm superior to the right zygoma and 1 cm anterior to the external auditory canal, extending across the midline 3 cm anterior to the coronal suture, and ending 4 cm superior to the zygoma and 1 cm anterior to the external auditory canal. The patient was prepped and draped in the standard sterile fashion.
2. (X cc) of local anesthetic (X% lidocaine and epinephrine at 1:X) was infiltrated along the line of the drawn incision. With a (10) blade and monopolar electrocautery, the scalp flap was reflected and retracted with skin hooks to expose 6 cm anterior and 3 cm posterior to the coronal suture.
3. A craniotomy 6 cm anterior and 2 cm posterior to the coronal suture, and 3 cm to the right and 2 cm to the left of the sagittal suture was performed after burr holes were placed at the described anterior and posterior margins.
4. The dura was irrigated and hemostasis was achieved with bipolar electrocautery. Strips of absorbable hemostatic matrix were placed at the edges of exposed dura, and 4-0 silk circumferential dural tenting sutures were placed.
5. The dura was elevated with a sharp hook/4-0 silk suture, and opened with a 15 blade. The incision was extended with long straight scissors and dural forceps in a U-shaped fashion based medially along the sagittal sinus. The dural flap was reflected over midline and the cortex was protected with a moist cotton dressing.
6. The arachnoid in the interhemispheric fissure was opened sharply with an 11 blade. The arachnoid adhesions between the hemisphere and sagittal sinus were divided with irrigating bipolar electrocautery. Small bridging veins were divided. The optimal trajectory to the lesion was identified with computer navigation.
7. The dissection was continued inferiorly along the falx. The pericallosal arteries were separated to each side. A 1 x 2–cm corpus callosotomy was

fashioned with irrigating bipolar electrocautery and suction, and the dissection was carried to the vessels of the ependymal lining, which were
cauterized. The ependymal layer was traversed and the brain retractor
was repositioned just beyond the inferior callosal margin.
8. Procedure varies.
9. Crani closure.

G. SUBOCCIPITAL APPROACH (CPT 61500 SERIES)

1. The head was placed in Mayfield-Kees three-point fixation and the
    patient was then rolled prone onto laminectomy rolls on the operating
    table. The table was placed and mild reverse Trendelenberg. The arms
    were tucked to the sides and head was positioned in capital flexion. All
    bony prominences and peripheral nerves were padded. The occipito-
    cervical area was shaved, then prepped and draped as usual.
2. (X cc) of local anesthetic (X% lidocaine and epinephrine at 1:X) was infil-
    trated along the line of the drawn incision. With a (10) blade and monopo-
    lar electrocautery, a skin incision was extended from just below the inion
    to the spinous process of C2. The dissection was carried down through
    the midline raphe to the occipital bone. Muscle and soft tissue were dis-
    sected in a subperiosteal manner from the occiput and C1 arch.
3. Burr holes were made on both sides of the midline 2/3 of the distance
    between the foramen magnum and inion. The underlying dura was sepa-
    rated from the inner table in each direction with a Penfield #3. Cuts were
    extended between the burr holes and also curving laterally and then infe-
    rior to the foramen magnum using a (B-1 drill with a foot plate). The bone
    flap was elevated and preserved in moist sponges.
4. The dura was irrigated and hemostasis was achieved with bipolar elec-
    trocautery. Strips of absorbable hemostatic matrix were placed at the
    edges of exposed dura.
5. The cervical dura was elevated with a (sharp hook/4-0 silk suture), and
    opened with an (11) blade. CSF was released, allowing the cerebellum
    to relax. The dura over the cerebellar hemispheres was similarly ele-
    vated and opened in a V-like fashion toward the midline falx cerebelli
    sinus, which was double clipped with Weck clips and transected. A (4-0
    Neurolon) was tied around the inferior aspect of the cerebellar sinus and
    the clip was removed. The incision was extended inferiorly, paralleling
    the falx sinus and connecting it with the opening in the cervical dura. The
    dura was then retracted with fine silk suture.
6. Procedure varies.
7. Crani closure (multiple layers, watertight dural closure).

H. RETROSIGMOID (RETROMASTOID) APPROACH (CPT 61500 SERIES)

1. The patient was placed in the supine position, with the head was placed in
    Mayfield-Kees three-point fixation. The head was turned to the (right) and
    parallel to the floor, with the chin tucked toward the chest. In this position,
    the (left) retromastoid area was brought to the center of the operative
    field. All bony prominences and peripheral nerves were padded.

2. The retromastoid area was shaved and prepped in the usual fashion. An operative site was marked along the plane from the left zygoma to the inion, denoting the transverse sinus, and along the plane of digastric groove intersecting this at a 70°, denoting the sigmoid sinus. A curvilinear incision was marked.

3. After subcutaneous infiltration of (1% lidocaine and epinephrine), the skin was incised with a (10 blade) and electrocautery. The underlying muscle was elevated. Self-retaining retractors were placed.

4. A single burr hole was fashioned at the junction between the transverse and sigmoid sinuses. A 4-cm rectangular bone flap was cut using a B-1 drill with a foot plate, and then elevated. The craniotomy was then enlarged laterally and superiorly with a Kerrison punch until the inferior edge of the transverse sinus and medial edge of the sigmoid sinus were exposed. Bone wax was applied for hemostasis and to occlude and open portion of the mastoid air cells.

5. The dura was irrigated and hemostasis was achieved with bipolar electrocautery. Strips of absorbable hemostatic matrix were placed at the edges of exposed dura. The dura was elevated with a sharp hook, and opened with an (11) blade. The incision was extended anteriorly to the junction of the transverse and sigmoid sinuses with Metzenbaum scissors and dural forceps.

6. Procedure varies.

7. Crani closure (multiple layers, watertight dural closure).

I. PRESIGMOID APPROACH (CPT 61500 SERIES)

1. The patient was positioned supine with the head placed in three-point fixation, turned to the (right) with the neck slightly flexed and the shoulder elevated on a bean bag. All bony prominences and peripheral nerves were padded. The head and neck in the right postauricular area, as well as the abdomen, were prepped and draped as usual. A planned curvilinear scalp incision was marked behind the ear, from the posterior temporal region to a point posteroinferior to the mastoid.

2. After subcutaneous infiltration with (1% lidocaine with epinephrine), a 3-cm linear incision was made on the abdomen. An adipose graft was harvested with scissors. The scalp site was then infiltrated with (1% lidocaine with epinephrine) and incised with a (10) blade and electrocautery. The muscle was elevated and self-retaining retractors were placed.

3. A partial mastoidectomy was begun at the asterion with superior and lateral extension into the mastoid air cells using a drill, and all exposed air cells were occluded with bone wax. The posterolateral portion of the petrous pyramid was removed and the sigmoid and distal transverse sinuses were skeletonized. The craniectomy was extended anterosuperior to the transverse-sigmoid sinus junction.

4. The dura was irrigated and hemostasis was achieved with bipolar electrocautery and absorbable hemostatic matrix. (4-0 Neurulon) circumferential dural tenting sutures were placed. The temporal dura was elevated with a sharp hook, and incised inferiorly with an 11 blade. The presigmoid dura was opened and the two incisions were connected anterior to the vein

of Labbé. The superior petrosal sinus was double ligated with Weck clips and transected. Under microscopy, the tentorium was divided toward the incisura.
5. Procedure varies.
6. Crani closure (multiple layers, watertight dural closure).

J. TRANSPETROSAL TRANSLABYRINTHINE APPROACH (CPT 61500 SERIES)

1. The head was then placed in three-point fixation, turned to the left side and elevated above the heart, with a roll under the right shoulder, so that the mastoid process was at the highest point in the operative field. All bony prominences and peripheral nerves were padded. The right temporal and retromastoid regions and the left lower quadrant of the abdomen were shaved, prepped, and draped sterilely. A planned horseshoe-shaped incision was drawn in the right temporo-suboccipital region, starting anterior to the right ear at the level of the zygoma, extending posterosuperiorly, and then curving inferiorly into the retromastoid region.

2. After subcutaneous infiltration with (1% lidocaine with epinephrine), a 3-cm linear incision was made in the abdomen. An adipose graft was harvested with scissors, and the wound was closed with running subcuticular absorbable suture. The scalp site was then infiltrated with 1% lidocaine with epinephrine and incised with a #10 blade and monopolar electrocautery. The temporalis was taken down with the scalp flap.

3. A mastoidectomy was begun at the asterion with superior and lateral extension into the mastoid air cells. The cortical bone was removed to the posterior wall of the external auditory canal. The sigmoid sinus was skeletonized inferiorly through the infralabyrinthine air cells to the jugular bulb. The semicircular canals were removed and the vestibule was opened to reveal the nerves to the lateral, inferior, and superior ampullae. The internal auditory canal and entire facial nerve were skeletonized. Bone was removed from the superior wall of the internal auditory canal. The malleus and incus were removed, obliterating the middle ear. The posterior temporal craniotomy was performed, and the petrous bone was drilled flat.

4. The dura of the posterior fossa in the presigmoid region was opened, and the dura of the subtemporal region was opened, basing it inferiorly.

5. Procedure varies.

6. The dura was closed with a synthetic graft for the supratentorial area. Autologous fat was used to close and seal the posterior fossa dura. The bone was replaced with titanium plates. Air cells were sealed with bone wax. The middle ear, internal auditory canal, and cavity created by the mastoidectomy were filled with fat.

7. Crani closure.

K. FAR LATERAL APPROACH (CPT 61500 SERIES)

1. The head was turned 90° to the left side. The neck was carefully inspected, revealing no jugular venous compression. The head was shaved, prepped, and draped in the usual sterile fashion. A planned retromastoid "field

hockey stick" incision was drawn, with lateral limb extending to just below the right mastoid process and medial limb to just below C3.

2. After subcutaneous infiltration with (1% lidocaine with epinephrine), a 3-cm linear incision was made in the abdomen. An adipose graft was harvested with scissors, and the wound was closed with running subcuticular absorbable suture. The scalp site was then infiltrated with (1% lidocaine and epinephrine) and incised with a (10) blade and monopolar electrocautery. The dissection was carried down through the subcutaneous and soft tissues, and the musculocutaneous flap was raised in one layer. The right vertebral artery was identified entering the dura above the C1 arch and preserved. The muscles were elevated off of the lateral mass of C1 and occipital condyle.

3. Using the pneumatic drill, a suboccipital craniotomy was performed, with the lip of the foramen magnum as an entry point. The craniotomy was extended superolaterally to expose the transverse and sigmoid sinuses down to the jugular bulb. The arch of C1 was then removed to the midline with Leksell rongeurs. Medial mobilization of the vertebral artery was achieved by drilling a notch on the portion of the arch beneath it. The medial third of the occipital condyle and lateral mass of C1 was then removed.

4. The dura was irrigated and hemostasis was achieved with bipolar electrocautery. Strips of absorbable hemostatic matrix were placed at the edges of absorbable dura.

5. The dura was elevated with a sharp hook/4-0 silk suture, and opened with a 11 blade. The incision was further opened with scissors into three lateral triangular leaves based on the transverse sinus, sigmoid sinus, and vertebral artery.

6. Procedure varies; e.g., tumor resection or aneurysm clipping.

7. Crani closure.

L. TRANSPHENOIDAL HYPOPHYSECTOMY (CPT 61548, 62165)

The transsphenoidal approach to the sella will be dictated in detail in a separate report by ENT attending. To summarize,

1. The central face and abdomen were prepped and draped, after injection of the palatal foramina with epinephrine. Sterile drapes were placed around the nasal area above the lip along the malar eminences. The eyes were carefully protected. The nares were treated with oxymetazoline spray/pledgets soaked in cocaine.

2. Assisted by a handheld speculum and computer navigation, an incision was made along the medial aspect of the mucosa, which was elevated off the right cartilaginous septum. The cartilaginous septum was separated from the bony septum, which was fractured to the patient's left side. (A small bone graft was obtained for reconstituting the sella later. The mucosa and vascular pedicle were preserved for a later mucosal flap).

3. The speculum was advanced to the anterior wall of the sphenoid sinus and the rostrum. Mucosal dissection was carried out and a self-retaining retractor was inserted. Under endoscopy/microscopy, a small opening through the anterior wall of the sphenoid sinus was made with rongeurs.

The sphenoid sinus mucosa was stripped with a pituitary rongeur. Hemostasis was achieved with gel hemostatic matrix.

4. The carotid arteries and sella midline were identified. A sphenoidotomy was made with a small osteotome and rongeurs or drill, and then widened bilaterally out to the lateral margins. The intersphenoid septi were removed and drill flushed back to the sella. The sella face was flattened and then opened with the drill. Bone over the face of sella was removed from the superior intracavernous sinus above, to the sella floor below, and also from the cavernous sinus on one side to the other.

5. Dura was incised in a (cruciate/trap door) fashion with a #11 blade. The tumor was identified and removed with gentle suction and ring curettes. The entire cavity was irrigated with antibiotic solution and lined with a layer of fibrillar absorbable hemostatic agent.

6. Attention was then directed to the subumbilical region which had been sterilely prepared. After subcutaneous infiltration with (1% lidocaine with epinephrine) and placement of a 1–1/2-in. curvilinear incision, subcutaneous fat was harvested with scissors. Hemostasis was obtained with electrocautery. The wound was irrigated with antibiotic solution and closed in layers with absorbable braided suture in the subcutaneous tissue and monofilament in the skin. A sterile dressing was applied. The fat graft was then carefully filled with fat.

7. The sella floor was reconstructed with a piece of (nasal cartilage/synthetic absorbable graft), over which lay the mucosal graft. This was covered with fibrin sealant and buttressed with gel hemostatic matrix externally. The septum and nasal mucosa were brought back to the midline. Pledgits were placed by ENT in the nasal cavity.

8. The nose and oropharynx were cleared of debris, the stomach and esophagus suctioned. All drapes were removed, and the patient was released from Mayfield-Kees fixation.

III. SPINE

Additional common CPT codes include use of bone graft (20930, 1, 6-8)

A. OCCIPITOCERVICAL FUSION (CPT 22590)

1. The head was placed in Mayfield-Kees three-point fixation and the patient was then rolled prone onto laminectomy rolls. Using fluoroscopy, the neck was aligned in a neutral position.

2. The hair was shaved in the occipitocervical area. The occipital cervical area was prepped and draped in the usual sterile fashion.

3. After subcutaneous infiltration with (1% lidocaine with epinephrine), a skin incision over the preoperatively marked site was made with a (10) blade, and the dissection was carried down through subcutaneous tissues to the occipital bone. Muscle and soft tissue was dissected off of the occiput, C1 arch, and C2 spinous process.

4. Under fluoroscopic guidance, bilateral (3.5 x 28) mm screws were placed into the lateral masses of C1 and bilateral (3.5 x 14) mm screws were

placed into the pars of C2. A (31) mm plate was anchored to the occiput with (4.8 x 8) mm and (4.8 x 10) mm screws. A (3.5 x 150) mm rod was cut, curved, and fashioned to attach to the occipital plate and cervical screws, giving rigid fixation.

5. We then used a pneumatic drill to carefully burr along the occiput and arches of C1 and C2. A combination of allograft, iliac crest graft, and blood were placed in and around the rod and fixation, directly on the burr sites. Strips of bone morphogenetic protein were laid over the bone grafts.

6. Spine closure.

B. ANTERIOR CERVICAL DISKECTOMY AND FUSION (CPT 63075, 22554, 22845, 20931)

1. In a supine position, the neck was slightly extended by placing a roll underneath the shoulders. Preoperative X-ray was taken to ensure the appropriate level and visualization. The anterior neck, upper chest, and lower jaw were prepped and draped as usual.

2. After subcutaneous infiltration with (1% lidocaine and epinepherine), a 5-cm transverse incision was made over the (right) anterior neck along the skin crease. The skin incision was carried down to divide the platysma. Subplatysmal flaps were raised cephalad and caudad with Metzenbaum scissor dissection.

3. Dissection was carried medial to the sternocleidomastoid muscle and carotid and jugular vein and lateral to the trachea and esophagus. The prevertebral space was entered through the anterior margin of the sternocleidomastoid, the upper half of the omohyoid, and the plane between the carotid artery and esophagus.

4. The prevertebral fascia was exposed and then opened up sharply, and the (C6–7) interspace was verified by a lateral X-ray of the cervical spine with an 18-gauge spinal needle put in disk space as a marker. Bilateral longus colli muscles were elevated and dissected from medial to lateral for wider exposure of the transverse distance of the disk space, and also for placement of the self-retaining retractor blade with teeth.

5. The disk space was then incised with a (15) blade. The anterior bone spurs were removed with an Adson rongeur. The disk space was widened using the vertebral body distractor. The anterior lip of (C6) was removed with a (3-mm) Kerrison rongeur. The disk space was curetted with an upgoing cup curette and then decorticated with a cutting burr. The posterior spurs were thinned down to expose more of the posterior longitudinal ligament. The ligament was dissected free from the underlying dura, and removed with a (2-mm) Kerrison rongeur. The residual posterior spurs were removed with a (2-mm) Kerrison rongeur. Hemostasis was obtained with (Company) matrix hemostatic sealant. The disk space was irrigated and measured.

6. A (lordotically) shaped bone plug (8 mm in height, 15 mm in width, and 12 mm in depth) was tapped into the (C6–C7) interspace.

7. A (16-mm) anterior plate was secured by two (X-mm) upper screws aimed superomedially into the (C6) body, and two lower screws aimed perpendicularly into the (C7) body. X-ray/fluoroscopy of the cervical spine revealed the implants were in excellent position.

8. After removal of the vertebral body distractor and self-retaining retractor, surrounding structures and vasculature were checked and were found intact. The wound was irrigated thoroughly with warm saline antibiotic solution, and further hemostasis was achieved with matrix hemostatic sealant and bipolar cautery.

9. The incision was closed with interrupted inverted (4-0 Vicryl) in the subcutaneous layer and (4-0 Monocryl) suture in the skin. The drapes were removed and sterile dressings were applied.

C. ANTERIOR CERVICAL CORPECTOMY, PLACEMENT OF INTERBODY CAGE (CPT 63081, 63082, 22851)

1. See anterior cervical discectomy and fusion (ACDF).

2. After placing two self-retaining retractors underneath the longus colli muscles, a vertebrectomy was performed at the (C4) level with a Leksell rongeur and high-speed drill. The posterior longitudinal ligament was identified.

3. A foraminotomy was achieved using the (x-mm) Kerrison punch. The endplates of the bottom of the (C3) and top of the (C5) levels were prepared using the curved curettes. The vertebral body space was carefully distracted.

4. We packed the previously measured mesh interbody cage with the cancellous bone chips, and placed it at the interbody space with careful tapping. The position of the cage was confirmed with intraoperative fluoroscopy.

5. Closure as previously described (see ACDF).

D. CERVICAL LAMINOPLASTY (CPT 63050)

1. The patient was placed into Mayfield-Kees three-point fixation and carefully turned prone onto laminectomy rolls. The neck was kept in a neutral position. All bony prominences and peripheral nerves were padded. The abnormal cervical level was identified fluoroscopically. The hair was shaved in the cervical midline, and then prepped and draped in the usual sterile fashion.

2. After subcutaneous infiltration with (1% lidocaine and epinephrine), a midline incision was made with a (10) blade and monopolar electrocautery. The dissection was carried down through the fascia in the midline, and the spinous processes of (C5–C7) were identified. The subperiosteal dissection of paraspinous muscles was carried out from (C5–C7), and the correct site was reidentified fluoroscopically.

3. A self-retaining retractor was placed. A portion of the (left) lateral laminae of (C6 and C7) was removed with a power drill. The remainder of the lamina and ligamentum were removed with curettes and fine Kerrison rongeurs. The dorsal portion of the lamina on the contralateral side was drilled down. A greenstick fracture of the contralateral lamina was performed and the other side was secured with (X) plates and screws.

4. Meticulous hemostasis was established from the epidural veins with bipolar electrocautery and gel hemostatic matrix.

5. Spine closure.

E. KYPHOPLASTY (CPT 22523 FOR THORACIC, 22524 FOR LUMBAR)

1. The patient was positioned on a Jackson table to allow for natural extension of the spine and facilitate fluoroscopy in multiple planes. Two C-arms were placed, one for the AP and one for lateral X-rays. The (level) was confirmed on multiple X-rays, and the appropriate incision site was drawn.

2. After subcutaneous infiltration of (1% lidocaine with epinephrine), a (X-gauge) needle was used to puncture the skin and facia, but was not advanced to the laminae. A stab incision was made and the first guide pin was used to penetrate the fractured vertebral body through an (extrapedicular/ transpedicular) approach under biplane fluoroscopic guidance.

3. A cannulated obturator was placed over the guide. A working cannula was placed over this and advanced until its tip was seated in the posterior portion of the vertebral body.

4. A hand-held drill was then advanced through the cannula anteromedially toward the anterior vertebral body cortex. The drill was removed from the cannula and replaced with an inflatable balloon tamp.

5. The tamp was advanced into the vertebral body and inflated to (X pressure), elevating the depressed end plates, thereby restoring the vertebral body height. The tamp was then withdrawn through the cannula.

6. Methyl methacrylate cement was prepared and, when it had a firm consistency, was injected into the cavity created by the inflation of the balloon tamp. The cavity was filled (2/3) of the way back to the posterior vertebral body cortex, as determined by fluoroscopy. No efflux of methyl methacrylate was identified at anytime.

7. The bone void filler tools and cannula were removed.

8. Spine closure.

F. LUMBAR LAMINECTOMY (WITH DISKECTOMY [CPT 63030]/WITH FORAMINOTOMY [CPT 63047])

1. The patient was carefully turned prone onto Jackson table with a radiolucent Wilson frame. All bony prominences and peripheral nerves were padded. The lumbar area was prepped and draped in the usual sterile fashion, and a (5-cm) midline incision was marked between the (L4 and L5) spinous processes, which were confirmed on fluoroscopy.

2. After subcutaneous infiltration with (1% lidocaine with epinephrine), the skin was opened with a (10) blade and monopolar electrocautery. A self-retaining retractor was placed. The lumbodorsal fascia was dissected in the midline to the tips of the spinous processes. The musculo-ligamentous tissues were elevated off of the spinous processes, and a subperiosteal dissection of the muscle and fascia was carried out with the assistance of Cobb dissectors. Deep self-retaining retractors were placed.

3. (The spinous processes of (L4 and L5) were removed with a Leksell ronguer). The interlaminar space was cleaned with a large straight curette. The lamina was freed from the ligamentum flavum with a small, upgoing curette, and then removed with (drill/Kerrison punch/Leksell rongeurs). The medial aspects of the facets were removed with (X mm) Kerrison

punch after thinning them with a high speed drill. The pedicles below were identified by palpation with a nerve hook.

4. The high speed drill and (X-mm) Kerrison punch were used to trim the inferior aspect of the (L4) lamina and the medial third of the inferior facet of (L4). A dissector was used to separate ligament from the bone. The (X-mm) Kerrison punch was used to remove the medial third of the superior facet of (L5). The trough was extended laterally to the left pedicle in the same manner.

5. The neural foramen was examined and (L5) nerve root compression was noted. The superior facet was punched out with a (X-mm) Kerrison rongeur inserted into the foramen. Nerve root decompression within the foramen was confirmed by palpation with a nerve hook. (An anti-inflammatory steroid was administered onto the nerve root.)

6. The (right L4) nerve root was retracted medially and the annulus fibrosis visualized. The annulus was incised with a #11 blade and disk fragments were brought into view with a nerve hook and then removed with a pituitary rongeur.

7. Epidural hemostasis was achieved by application of gel hemostatic matrix.

8. Spine closure.

IV. CAROTID ENDARTERECTOMY (CPT 35301)

1. The patient was placed supine and the head was turned 20° to the (left). The (right) aspect of the neck was prepped and draped in the usual sterile manner.

2. After subcutaneous infiltration with (1% lidocaine with epinephrine), a 8 cm skin incision extending from 1 cm posterior to the angle of the mandible to the anterior border of the sternocleidomastoid was made with a (10) blade and monopolar electrocautery.

3. The platysma was divided and the carotid sheath entered proximal to the carotid bifurcation. The internal jugular vein was identified and the dissection was continued medial. The facial vein was double-ligated and transected.

4. (The carotid bifurcation was instilled with 0.3 cc 1% lidocaine without epinephrine). The external carotid artery was isolated, and its proximal branches were temporarily occluded with (temporary aneurysm clips). Silastic loops were placed around the common and internal carotid arteries. Mild hypertension was induced and an IV bolus of 5000 units heparin was administered. (Aneurysm clips) were placed sequentially on the internal and external carotid arteries. (A Fogarty clip) was then placed on the common carotid artery.

5. A common carotid arteriotomy was made with a (15) blade, and then extended into the internal carotid artery beyond the plaque with Potts scissors. The plaque was circumferentially bluntly dissected from the underlying media to a point distal to normal intima within the internal carotid artery. The field was irrigated with heparinized saline.

6. The distal portion of the arteriotomy was closed with (running 5–0 poly-propylene suture) with bites 2 mm from the sewn edge to approximately midpoint on the incision, and a separate running suture was begun from the proximal end of the incision. Back bleeding of the internal and common carotid arteries was allowed for several seconds, and then the sutures were tightened and secured to each other.

7. The clips were sequentially removed from the external and common carotid arteries, allowing debris to be flushed into the external system. Then the clip was removed from the internal carotid. There was no evidence of bleeding from the suture line.

8. The incision was closed with (interrupted 3-0 absorbable braided suture) in the platysma, (interrupted inverted 4-0 absorbable braided suture) in the subcutaneous layer, and (4-0 monocryl suture) in the skin. Sterile dressings were applied and the drapes removed.

V. PERIPHERAL NERVE

A. SURAL NERVE/GASTROCNEMIUS MUSCLE BIOPSY (CPT 64795)

1. The patient was placed in the (supine/prone) position. The (right) lateral ankle and leg were prepped and draped in the usual sterile fashion. A planned (3-cm) vertical linear incision midway between the Achilles tendon and lateral malleolus was marked. A second (3-cm) vertical incision on the lateral aspect of the gastrocnemius muscle was marked.

2. Without local anesthetic, an incision was made beginning at the ankle and carried with sharp dissection through Scarpa's fascia.

3. The lesser saphenous vein was identified, and the sural nerve was found deep and posterior to this.

4. The sural nerve was further exposed by dissection beyond the distal and proximal incision margins, and local anesthetic was injected into the nerve proximal to the planned nerve division site.

5. The nerve was divided beyond the incision margins to avoid subsequent neuroma formation. A (X-cm) long nerve specimen was resected, and the nerve specimen was submitted for pathologic evaluation. The incision was closed with interrupted inverted (4-0 absorbable braided) suture in the subcutaneous layer and running (4-0 absorbable) subcuticular suture in the skin. A sterile dressing was applied.

6. Without local anesthetic, an incision was made on the posterior lateral leg and carried with sharp dissection through Scarpa's fascia. Several strips of muscle oriented in the long axis of the muscle bundle were isolated from the surrounding tissues and sharply excised. These (X-cm) specimens were also sent for pathologic evaluation.

7. The incision was closed with interrupted inverted (4-0 absorbable braided) suture in the subcutaneous layer and running (4-0 absorbable) subcuticular suture in the skin. A sterile dressing was applied. The drapes were removed.

B. CARPAL TUNNEL RELEASE (CPT 64721)

1. The patient was positioned supine with (his/her) (right) arm extended, hand supinated, and digits extended in a (wrist/hand brace). The entire hand up to the elbow was prepped and draped in the usual sterile fashion. A planned (3–4-cm) incision was marked, extending from the distal wrist crease at a point medial to the palmaris longus tendon, to a point on the palm just ulnar to the volar crease.

2. After subcutaneous infiltration of (1% lidocaine without epinephrine), the skin was opened with a (15) blade and dissected to the subcutaneous fat. Two small self-retaining retractors were placed at successively greater depths as the skin and subcutaneous tissues were cut for better exposure.

3. The fibers of the Palmaris longus tendon and the palmar aponeurosis were divided, exposing the subjacent flexor retinaculum. The flexor retinaculum was cut longitudinally with a (11) blade. A #4 Penfield dissector was placed under the retinaculum to protect the structures below, as the retinaculum was cut further in a proximal to distal direction.

4. The blunt end of a Senn retractor was used to retract the skin upward to expose the retinaculum proximally under the wrist. Small, blunt scissors were then used to cut the retinaculum proximally to where it merged with the distal forearm antebrachial fascia. The median nerve was well visualized and relieved from its compression in the carpal tunnel.

5. The wound was irrigated with warm saline and hemostasis was achieved with bipolar electrocautery.

6. The skin edges were re-approximated with (4-0 nylon vertical mattress) suture. Sterile dressings were applied and the drapes were removed.

VI. CRANIOSYNOSTOSIS REPAIR

A. METOPIC SYNOSTECTOMY (CPT 61550)

1. The patient was placed supine. The entire head was shaved and positioned on a padded gel horseshoe headrest with a roll beneath the shoulders. Sterile corneal shields were placed after placing ophthalmic antibiotic ointment over the cornea. The endotracheal tube was protected by a Mayo stand, and the upper face and head were prepped and draped in the usual sterile fashion. A bicoronal Z-plasty incision was marked.

2. After subcutaneous infiltration of (1% lidocaine without epinephrine), the skin was opened with a (15) blade and monopolar electrocautery. The scalp was elevated with skin hooks, and the dissection was carried down to the supraorbital rims and lateral supraorbital segments bilaterally.

3. The pericranium was incised behind the coronal sutures and above the attachment of the temporalis muscle to the lateral edge of the orbital rim. The pericranium was freed around the anterior fontanelle and elevated off of the frontal bone, down to the supraorbital rims. The supraorbital nerves were mobilized along with the periorbita by cutting the supraorbital

foramen with a small osteotome. The temporalis muscles were freed from their fossae, exposing the squamosal sutures.

4. Using a pneumatic power drill, burr holes were made over the metopic suture, in addition to the bilateral pterions. A bifrontal craniotomy was completed with the drill, crossing the midline posteriorly behind the coronal sutures and anteriorly along the supraorbital bar. The bone flap was elevated and removed with an Obwegeser elevator. A tongue-and-groove cut was performed within the temporal regions for extension of the supraorbital bar into the temporal fossae. The inner table was thinned in the area of the thickened metopic suture, allowing maintenance of the supraorbital bar extended to the frontonasal suture.

5. The periorbita was dissected from inside of the orbital roof. Malleable retractors were placed into the orbit and also used to lightly retract the frontal dura. The orbital roof was cut behind the orbital rims bilaterally, extending to the lateral posts. The orbital bar was greenstick fractured anteriorly, normalizing the supraorbital region. The frontal area, which was reshaped using a Tessier form, was reattached to the frontal bar with absorbable plates and screws, reconstructing the forehead. The orbital rim and frontal bone were recontoured to a normal shape.

6. The pericranium was repositioned and anchored with interrupted 4-0 absorbable braided suture. The temporalis muscle was mobilized and reattached to the bone and absorbable plating system in the temporal regions.

7. The incisions were irrigated with warm saline, and then closed with (interrupted inverted 4-0 absorbable braided suture) in the subcutaneous layer and (4-0 nylon suture in the skin). The drapes were removed, sterile dressings were applied, and a stocking cap was placed.

B. BICORONAL SYNOSTECTOMY (CPT 61550)

1. The patient was placed in the supine position on the operating table. The entire head was shaved. The patient was carefully positioned on a padded gel horseshoe headrest with a roll beneath the shoulders. The endotracheal tube was protected by a Mayo stand, and then the upper face and head were prepped and draped in the usual sterile fashion. A bicoronal Z-plasty incision was marked.

2. After subcutaneous infiltration of (1% lidocaine without epinephrine), the skin was opened with a (15) blade and monopolar electrocautery. The scalp was elevated with skin hooks, and the dissection was carried down to the supraorbital rims and lateral supraorbital segments bilaterally, the frontonasal and frontozygomatic suture, and to the temporal fossa.

3. (Right/left/both) coronal sutures were found to be closed. The pericranium was incised behind the coronal sutures and above the attachment of the temporalis muscle to the lateral edge of the orbital rim. The pericranium was freed around the anterior fontanelle and elevated off of the frontal bone, down to the orbital rim.

4. A line representing the orbital bandeau was drawn (1 cm) above both orbits. A bifrontal craniotomy extending beyond the coronal sutures was

also marked. Using a pneumatic power drill, a burr hole was made in the midline at the metopic suture above the bandeau, in addition to the bilateral pterions. Using the anterior fontanelle as the access point, a bifrontal craniotomy was completed with the drill, and the bone flap was elevated and removed with an Obwegeser elevator.

5. The periorbita was dissected from inside of the orbital roof, and the frontonasal and frontozygomatic sutures were exposed. Malleable retractors were placed into the orbit and also used to lightly retract the frontal dura. With the pneumatic power drill, a cut was made in the orbital roofs bilaterally, as well in the region of the frontonasal sutures and across the frontozygomatic sutures. The frontozygomatic sutures were elevated with a small osteotome, freeing the frontal bars.

6. The frontal bar was reattached with absorbable plates and screws. The frontal and temporal bones, which were reconstructed and freed down to the squamosal suture, were reshaped and reattached to the frontal bar with absorbable plates and screws, reconstructing the orbital rims, forehead, and temporal fossa.

7. Closure as above.

C. SAGITTAL SYNOSTECTOMY (CPT 61550)

1. Patient was carefully turned prone onto a padded pediatric gel horseshoe headrest with the head slightly extended. All bony prominences, face, and peripheral nerves were padded and he was covered to maintain body warmth. In the usual sterile fashion, the head was prepped and draped from the anterior fontanelle to the lambda, and a planned biparietal/ sagittal/ Z-plasty incision was marked.

2. After subcutaneous infiltration of (1% lidocaine without epinephrine), the skin was opened with a (15) blade and monopolar electrocautery. The scalp was elevated with skin hooks, retracted with fine sutures, and dissected to (2.5 cm) on either side of midline.

3. The soft tissue surrounding the anterior fontanelle was freed with an Obwegeser, and the periosteum was incised sagittally on both sides (1.5 cm) lateral to the closed sagittal suture, to the level of the open lambdoid sutures.

4. Using a power drill, small burr holes were made in each lambdoid suture (1.5 cm) lateral to midline. Using a Lempert rongeur, the burr holes were connected by removing bone anteromedially up to the closed posterior portion of the sagittal suture. Using a power drill, the burr holes were then connected to the anterior fontanelle and coronal suture by two linear sagittal cuts placed (1.5 cm) to each side of the closed sagittal suture. The resulting bone flap was elevated off of the underlying dura and sagittal sinus with a #3 Penfield.

5. In the occipital area, the remaining lambdoid suture was removed with a rongeur. Using the pneumatic power drill, multiple barrel stave osteotomies were placed in the occipital bone extending toward the transverse sinuses. The bone was greenstick fractured outward, enlarging the occip-

ital region. Hemostasis was achieved with bipolar electrocautery, bone
wax, and gel hemostatic matrix.

6. In the same fashion, multiple barrel stave osteotomies were placed in
the parietal bones bilaterally, which were greenstick fractured to enlarge
and reshape the parietal areas. Sharp areas of bone were removed with a
rongeur and contoured to a rounder shape.

7. Closure as above.

DISCHARGE SUMMARY

1. Your first and last name (spell out)
2. Patient's first and last name (spell out)
3. Medical record number
4. Attending physician's first and last name (spell out)
5. Type of report (Discharge Summary)
6. Date of service
7. Service (Neurosurgery/Neurology)
8. (Billing number)
9. Date of admission
10. Date of discharge
11. Primary diagnosis
12. Secondary diagnosis
13. Procedures (date, name, individual performing the procedure)
14. Consultations (Service, Attending)
15. Reason for admission (HPI)
16. Hospital course (by systems or date)
17. Disposition (home, rehab, other facility)
18. Diagnoses/status
19. Condition
20. Diet
21. Activity
22. Medications (name, dose, duration)
23. Follow up
24. Instructions/precautions (take off dressing, no swimming/bathing/show-
ering for (X) days, no heavy lifting > 10 lbs, return to clinic or call (e.g.,
fever > 101.4, erythema/edema/discharge from wound, new/worsening
neurological symptoms, uncontrolled pain, etc.)

III. NEURO CRITICAL CARE

Michael SB Edwards, MD

CHAPTER 19 ■ ANATOMY

Andrew Phelps, MD
NOTE: All figures in this chapter are courtesy of A. Phelps, MD

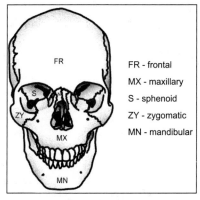

FR - frontal
MX - maxillary
S - sphenoid
ZY - zygomatic
MN - mandibular

Figure 19-1 Skull Frontal View

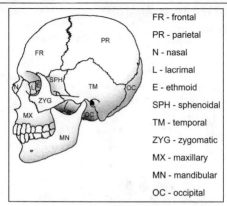

FR - frontal
PR - parietal
N - nasal
L - lacrimal
E - ethmoid
SPH - sphenoidal
TM - temporal
ZYG - zygomatic
MX - maxillary
MN - mandibular
OC - occipital

Figure 19-2 Skull Lateral View

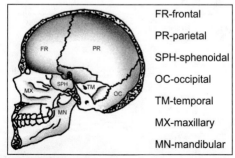

FR-frontal
PR-parietal
SPH-sphenoidal
OC-occipital
TM-temporal
MX-maxillary
MN-mandibular

Figure 19-3 Sagittal Skull Interior

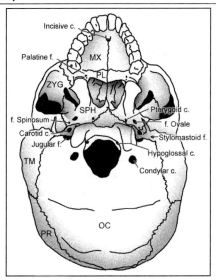

Figure 19-4 Skull Base Exterior, Inferior View

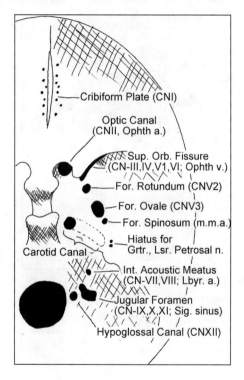

Figure 19-5 Skull Base, Interior View

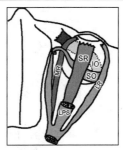

Figure 19-6 Extraocular Muscles

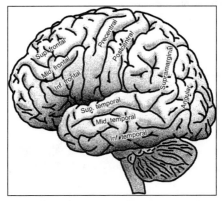

Figure 19-7 Cerebral Cortex, Lateral View

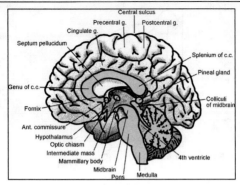

Figure 19-8 Cerebral Anatomy, Sagittal

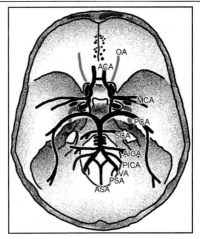

Figure 19-9 Circle of Willis (from above)
ACA = anterior cerebral artery; AICA = anterior inferior cerebellar artery;
ASA = anterior spinal artery; MCA = middle cerebral artery; OA = ophthalmic
artery; PCA = posterior cerebral artery; PICA = posterior inferior cerebellar
artery; PSA = posterior spinal artery; SCA = superior cerebellar artery;
VA = vertebral artery

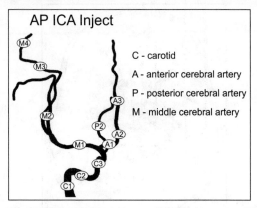

Figure 19-10 Angiogram of Internal Cerebral Artery (ICA) Injection, Anterior-Posterior (AP) View

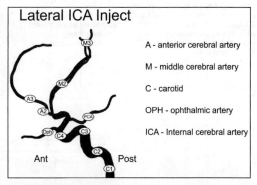

Figure 19-11 Angiogram of Internal Carotid Artery Injection, Lateral View

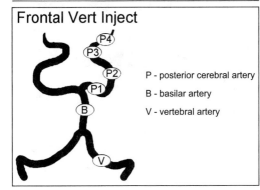

Figure 19-12 Angiogram of Vertebral Artery Injection, Frontal View

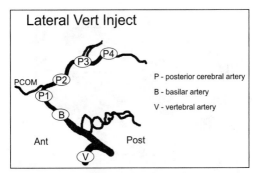

Figure 19-13 Angiogram of Vertebral Artery Injection, Lateral View

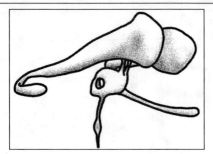

Figure 19-14 Ventricles

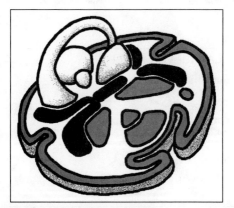

Figure 19-15 Basal Ganglia and Ventricular Anatomy

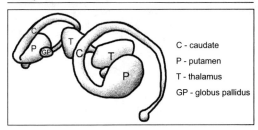

Figure 19-16 Basal Ganglia

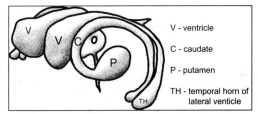

Figure 19-17 Putamen, Caudate

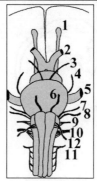

Figure 19-18 Brainstem Cranial Nerves, Ventral View

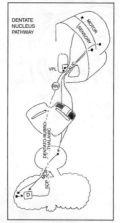

Figure 19-19 Dentate Nucleus Pathway
ALIC = anterior limb of internal capsule; D = dentate nucleus; MCP = middle
cerebellar peduncle; RN = red nucleus; SCP = superior cerebellar peduncle;
VPL = ventral posterolateral nucleus of the thalamus

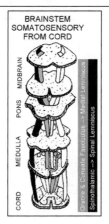

Figure 19-20 Brainstem Pathways Somatosensory

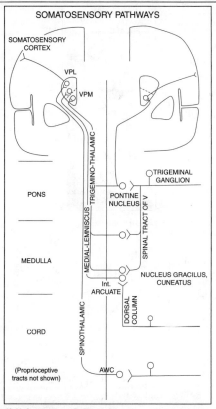

Figure 19-21 Somatosensory Pathways
AWC = anterior white commissure; VPL = ventral posterolateral nucleus of the thalamus; VPM = ventral posteromedial nucleus of the thalamus

CHAPTER 20 ■ ICU BASICS

Melanie G. Hayden Gephart, MD, MAS
Gregory Kapinos, MD, MS

Table 20-1 Blood Products

Product	Vol (ml)	Indications	Comments
Whole blood (WB)	400–500	• Massive transfusion in acute blood loss	• RBCs plus plasma • Rarely used
Packed red blood cells (PRBCs) See next page for specific types	250–350	• Increase O_2-carrying capacity if evidence/risk of end organ ischemia • Maintain volume and O_2 capacity in acute blood loss • **Not** indicated solely to maintain "target" Hb/Hct or for volume repletion (isovolemic anemia well tolerated if no cardiac, pulmonary, or cerebrovascular disease)	• Massive transfusion may cause hypothermia, low Ca^{++}, high K^+, dilutional thrombocytopenia • In critically ill patients, "restrictive" transfusion practice (i.e., at Hb of 7–9 mg/dl vs 10–12 mg/dl) may reduce mortality[2] • In acute MI, transfusion to Hct 30–33% may reduce mortality[3]
Platelet concentrates (PCs)	200–250 (per 5–6 unit pool)	• Bleeding and plts < 100K • Procedure and plts < 50K • Prophylactic if and plts < 10K • Bleeding and qualitatively abnormal platelets (e.g. uremia, ASA) • Serious bleeding after GP $II_b III_a$ inhibitor therapy	• 6-unit pool should raise count 50-60 K, less if alloimmunized. • May support platelets if refractory to SDPs • Contraindicated in consumptive coagulopathy (HIT, HUS/TTP, HELLP)
Single-donor platelets (SDPs)	200–250	• Same as platelet concentrates but fewer donor exposures (alloimmunization, infection)	• No data to support routine use to prevent alloimmunization[4]

(continued)

Table 20-1 (Continued)

Product	Vol (ml)	Indications	Comments
Fresh frozen plasma (FFP)	200–250	• Bleeding if multiple factor deficiency (massive transfusion, liver disease) • Disseminated intravascular coagulation or Thrombotic thrombocytopenic purpura • Reversal of warfarin • Factor XI deficiency	• Contains factors II, VII, IX, X, XI, XII, and XIII • Dose: 15 ml/kg for massive transfusion, 3-5 ml/kg to reverse warfarin (titrate to PT)
Cryoprecipitate	100–200 (per 10-unit pool)	• Replacement of fibrinogen when acutely depleted (< 100 mg/dl) or qualitatively abnormal • Serious bleeding after thrombolytic therapy • Factor VIII or vWF replacement if concentrate not available	• Contains factor VIII, vWF, fibronectin and fibrinogen • Fibrinogen in 10-unit pool = 4 units FFP (but roughly 20% of the volume)

Sources: Churchill[1], Hebert, et al[2], Wu, et al[3], TRAPS Group[4]

Table 20-2 Transfusion Risks

Adverse Outcome *	Risk per Unit Transfused
Hepatitis B	1: 220,000
Hepatitis C	1: 872,000–1,700,000
HTLV 1 or 2	1: 600,000
HIV 1 or 2	1: 1,400,000–2,400,000
Bacterial contamination – platelets / RBC	1: 2,000–3,000 / 1: 7,000–31,000
Fatal hemolytic transfusion reaction	1: 500,000
Fatal acute lung injury (ARDS)	1: 3,000,000
Mistransfusion	1: 14,000

* Emerging risks include variant CJD, West Nile virus, *T. cruzi*, malaria, babesiosis

Table 20-3 Normal Wound Healing Indices

Normal Wound Healing Indices	Malnutrition/Poor Wound Healing
Serum albumin > 3.5 g/dl	Total lymphocyte count < 1500/mm³
Absolute lymphocyte count > 1500/mm³	Serum albumin < 3.5 gm/dL
Absolute Doppler pressure 70 mmHg	Serum transferrin level < 226 mg/dL
Differential pressure index (ABI) > 0.5	
TcpO₂ 30 mm Hg	

Table 20-4 Relative Action of Vasopressors

Drug	Receptor	HR	Inotropy	SVR	Comments
Dopamine - *Low dose*	DA	0	0	↔↓	Renal and splanchnic vasodilatation
Dopamine - *High dose*	$\beta_1 \rightarrow \alpha_1$	↑	↑↑	↑↑	First-line pressor for SBP 70–90 mmHg
Dobutamine	$\beta_1, \beta_2 > \alpha_1$	↔↑	↑↑	↓↓	Inotrope and vasodilator; may lower BP
Norepinephrine	$\alpha_1, \alpha_2, \beta_1$	↔↑	↑↑	↑↑↑	For hypotension ref-ractory to dopamine; initial choice in sepsis
Epinephrine	α_1, α_2 β_1, β_2	↑↑	↑↑↑	↑↑↑	For refractory cardiac failure (e.g., post CABG) or anaphylaxis
Phenylephrine	α_1	0	0	↑↑↑	For refractory hypotension, esp. vasculogenic
Isoproterenol	β_1, β_2	↑↑↑	↑↑	↔↓	Primarily increases HR. May cause reflex hypotension
Vasopressin	V1a	0	0	↑↑	Despite acidosis

OCCULT CAUSES OF FEVER IN ICU PATIENTS[5,6]

- Infected IV catheters
- Drug reaction
- Otitis media, sinusitis (especially with nasogastric tube)
- Pulmonary embolism, deep vein thrombosis (DVT)
- Pancreatitis, acalculous cholecystitis
- *C. diff* colitis
- Fungal or secondary infection
- Central fever in head injury

CHECKLIST FOR PROPHYLAXIS

- DVT prophylaxis with low molecular weight heparin and sequential compression device (SCDs)
- GI ulcer prevention with proton pump inhibitor
- Enteral nutrition, when appropriate
- Wake Up & Breath: Once patient stable, daily withhold of sedation and mechanical ventilation (MV), unless proven dangerous. (ICP crises).

Indeed, spontaneous breathing trials and awakenings on a daily basis are the most effective treatment in the ICU to shorten days of MV, length of ICU and hospital stay and improve functional outcome and survival. (Girard TD, et al. Lancet 2008;371:126–34)

- Physical and occupational therapy to start as early as possible

VENTILATOR BASICS

WHEN TO INTUBATE

- Airway protection
- Severe facial trauma
- Preoperative for surgery
- Neurologic decline (GCS 8 or less)
- Pulmonary insufficiency (hypoventilation, hypoxemia, respiratory rate (RR) > 40, $PaO_2 < 60$)

HOW TO REPORT VENT SETTINGS

Mode, set rate, set tidal volume or set pressure support, set inspiratory/expiratory times, set positive end-expiratory pressure, set fractional inspired oxygen.

Then report observed respiratory rate, observed tidal volume, observed minute ventilation, abnormal breathing loops or patterns (stacking up breaths, no overbreathing, etc) and measured peak inspiratory pressure.

Initial ventilator settings: RR 12, TV = 7–10mL/kg or PS 10, PEEP 5, FiO_2 100% then titrate down to 30%.

- Determines ventilation ($paCO_2$): RR, TV (minute ventilation as a multiplication)
- Determines oxygenation (paO_2): PEEP, FiO_2

▨ Mode

Synchronized intermittent mandatory ventilation (SIMV) Patient determines volume of breaths over set rate

- Pressure support allows patient to overcome resistance of ventilator tubing

Continuous positive airway pressure (CPAP) PEEP, no rate, and no pressure support

- Same as spontaneous breathing trial (SBT)

BiPAP: Pressure support + PEEP without rate

Airway pressure release ventilation (APRV): Cycles between two different levels of CPAP (upper and lower)

- Baseline airway pressure is the upper CPAP level, intermittently released to a lower level

Continuous Mandatory Ventilation (CMV): Ventilator delivers breaths at preset intervals irrespective of patient effort

Assist Control (AC): Patient triggers the ventilator to deliver the full set tidal volume (VT) (above set rate)

▨ Fractional Inspired Oxygen (FiO₂)

- Room air = 21%
- Oxygen toxicity occurs at > 60%
- Start at 100% and titrate upon result of ABG

* Tidal volume (TV): Ideal = 7–10 mL/kg
- Lung protection: TV < 6 mL/kg IBW
- Intraoperative = 10–15 mL/kg
- High TV leads to barotrauma and high peak inspiratory pressures (PIP) (> 30)
  * Rate starts at 8–12, hyperventilation at 16–20
  * Positive End-Expiratory Pressure (PEEP)
- To prevent alveolar collapse
- Standard is 5, raise by 2 up to 15 cmH$_2$O when needed, in parallell with FiO$_2$
- Increasing PEEP decreases venous return
  * Arterial Blood Gacs (ABG)
- Report as pH/PaCO$_2$/PaO$_2$/bicarb/base excess
- PaO2 reflects oxygenation, PaCO$_2$ reflects ventilation
- Order daily and prn for intubated patients
  * Recruitment Maneuvers
- Set rate at 12 and TV at 7mL/kg, then increase PEEP to 20 cmH$_2$O for 20 sec only

▦ Rate
Start at 8–12

▦ Positive End-Expiratory Pressure (PEEP)
To prevent alveolar collapse
- Standard is five, raise by two to three when needed
- Increasing PEEP decreases venous return

▦ Arterial Blood Gas (ABG)
Report as pH/PaCO2/PaO2/bicarb/base excess
- PaO2 reflects oxygenation, PaCO2 reflects ventilation
- Order daily and prn for intubated patients

▦ Recruitment Procedures
Give large breath then increase PEEP

ACUTE RESPIRATORY DISTRESS SYNDROME (ARDS)
Hypoxemia refractory to increased FiO2
- Give small tidal volume (6mL/kg), high rate, high PEEP (8–10), keep PIP < 35, time-controlled pressure ventilation modify inspiratory to expiratory time ratio (normal is 1:2)

NEUROGENIC PULMONARY EDEMA
Fulminant, diffuse pulmonary edema, decreased compliance (requiring high positive end–expiratory pressure), and hypoxemia (requires increased FiO2)
- May involve circulating catecholamines or increased peripheral vascular resistance

▦ When to Extubate
- Tobin index = rapid shallow breathing index (RSBI): Respiratory rate/tidal volume (L). If RSBI > 105, 80% chance of respiratory failure after extubation
- Negative Inspiratory Force should be at least be –20 to –30 cm H2O
- Minute ventilation (MV) (MV = RR * TV) of > 8 L/min

- Improving clinical status
- ABG appropriate during spontaneous breathing trial
- Pass SBT
- Cuff leak test on patients with concern for edema (e.g., long cases prone with large blood loss)
- Cough

TREATMENT OF INCREASED INTRACRANIAL PRESSURE

- Sedation, head of bed at 30 degrees
- Cervical collar release and slight head turn opposite to main draining jugular
- Adjust minute ventilation for goal etCO2/PaCO2 30-35mmHg, (below will likely trigger ischemia, above will likely exacerbate ICP)
- Ventriculostomy or evacuation of the mass lesion if possible, along with medical osmotherapy (Mannitol 1g/kg x1 dose, then 23% hypertonic saline 30mL amp x1-4doses until ICP < 15)
- If recurrent crises, Mannitol 0.5g/kg q6h alternating with 3% saline 250mL q6h, with goal SerOsm > 320 and Na > 155
- Therapeutic hypothermia
- Bilateral hemicraniectomy and vertical bed
- Barbiturate coma with goal ICP < 15 (do not target BSP)
- Paralysis or abdominal decompressive laparotomy—last resort

COMA

Table 20-5 Adult Glasgow Coma Scale (GCS)

Eye (E)	Verbal (V)	Motor (M)
1—no eye opening	1—makes no sounds	1—no movements
2—opens eyes to painful stimuli	2—incomprehensible sounds	2—extensor posturing
3—opens eyes to voice	3—inappropriate words	3—flexor posturing
4—opens eyes spontaneously	4—confused, disoriented	4—move limbs away from the pain
	5—oriented, converses normally	5—grabs the hand afflicting pain
	T—if the patient is intubated	6—follows commands

NOTE: Consider the three values separately and in sum. The lowest possible GCS (sum) is 3, the highest is 15.TBI is classified as severe, with GCS <or= 8, moderate, GCS 9-12, and minor, GCS >or= 13.
SOURCE: Courtesy of G Kapinos, adapted from Teasdale et al. Lancet 1974;2:81–4.

HERNIATION SYNDROMES

Cingulate: Cingulate gyrus under the falx → anterior cerebral artery compression and stroke → leg weakness/paralysis

Uncal: Uncus of medial temporal lobe under the tentorial incisure → CN III and midbrain compression → dilated pupil and coma

Central: Diencephalon under the tentorial incisure → compression of the thalamus, midbrain → coma

Tonsillar: Cerebellar tonsils through the foramen magnum → compression of the medulla → cardiorespiratory arrest

Upward: Cerebellar parenchyma cephalad through incisura → kinking of the posterior cerebral artery, displacement of fourth ventricle

DETERMINATION OF BRAIN DEATH (> 5 YEARS OF AGE)

(1) **Indisputable context**: Patient suffered a severe brain injury, notorious for leading to diffuse neuronal loss due to primary or secondary processes (global ischemic or hemorrhagic insult, or possibly a focal lesion, but large enough to induce severe ICP elevation, or centered in the brainstem, destroying ascending activating pathways) E.g. cardiac arrest, drowning, large ischemic or hemorrhagic stroke, severe TBI, meningoencephalitis, protracted super-refractory convulsive status epilepticus, pontine neoplasm, etc. But patients found down unresponsive, with no clear context or no clear cause for coma, are not candidates until metabolic, endocrinologic and toxic causes are ruled out.

(2) **Severe neurologic insult** is objectivated: clinical devastation is documented and neuroimaging pattern corroborates the findings (e.g. diffuse SAH, large ICH, malignant infarct or edema, midline shift and herniation, or brainstem irreversible lesion).

(3) Condition deemed **irreversible**: it is not an ischemic lesion but a completed infarct, not a resorbable small hematoma or contusion, not in coma solely due to transient elevated ICP, not an inflammatory, toxic or metabolic insult, but a true tissue destruction.

(4) No concomitant process that can ensue unresponsiveness (on its own or by exacerbating the neuronal dysfunction due to the primary insult), i.e. **no confounding factor**: no recent use of sedative or paralytic drug, no severe hypothermia (<36 degrees Celsius), no severe hypotension, no extreme acid-base or metabolic abnormality, no known severe endocrinologic derangement.

(5) Clinical exam demonstrates deep coma (**no cortical response**): upon sternal rub and trapezius pinching, as well as retromandibular and supraorbital compression (to stimulate above any potential spinal cord injury level), patient exhibits no grimace and no motor response in 4 limbs (NB: brainstem reflexic movements like flexor and extensor posturing are signs of brainstem activity, ruling out brain death, but spinal reflexic movements like Lazarus or thumb-up sign in upper limbs and triple flexion in lower limbs are seen in brain death).

(6) Clinical exam demonstrates **no brainstem function**: dilated (4-9mm) pupils nonreactive to light, no corneal reflex, no oculocephalogyric reflex (cannot be performed if in neck collar), no caloric oculovestibular

reflex in each ear (cannot be performed if temporal bone fracture is documented or with otorrhagia), no pharyngeal or gag reflex with tongue depressor, no cough reflex upon tracheal suctioning, and apnea is seen upon 30sec of spontaneous ventilation mode (NB: documented context of facial or cervical trauma precludes full assessment of brainstem reflexes and leads to complementary paraclinical testing).

(7) Apnea test confirms **no respiratory drive** (loss of rudimentary medullary function): preoxygenate with 100% O2 for 10 min, send baseline ABG, place nasal cannula with O2 at 4–8 L/min in the disconnected ETT, monitor for 8-15min and abort if saturation ≤90%, arrhythmia or significant hypotension occurs. Look closely for respiratory movements. Positive apnea test is evidenced by no chest or abdomen excursions seen or felt throughout the 8–15min test, with final ABG documenting PaCO2 ≥ 60mmHg or a rise of ≥20mmHg from the initial ABG PaCO2, or pH ≤7.20 (confirming we reached extreme stimulation of the medulla that should have triggered agonal breaths). NB: patient is immediately reconnected to ventilator upon completion of this test, positive or negative, and is kept on artificial support in both outcomes.

(8) In case of significant facial or cervical trauma, clinical determination cannot be complete. Imaging is used to document these injuries (facial or cranial base fractures, cervical cord injury or cervical instability). In these traumatic cases, or if apnea test was aborted or inconclusive, and if patient's exam is otherwise suggestive of complete and irreversible loss of cerebral (cortical and brainstem) function, complementary **ancillary testing** may be useful. Choose 1 modality, as they are often inconsistent: EEG (looking for electrical silence), nuclear scan (looking for absence of metabolically-driven perfusion), cerebral angiography, CTA, MRI/MRA, or TCD (all looking for no flow in the circle of Willis).

(9) There is no need for 2 clinical evaluations distinct in time, but usually 2 separate attendings need to document **one evaluation** (clinical + apnea test) to determine brain death. Check with your particular hospital policy and state law.

(10) Once patient is declared, **continue support**, engage the organ donation network, coordinate pastoral care. If organ donation is not rejected by the family, patient/corpse will be kept on artificial support (not "life support" but "organ support") to promote organ physiological functions until harvesting/transplant, with homeostasis and adequate perfusion. In case of refusal of organ/tissue donation by the family, patient/corpse is then liberated from all lines and monitors, then disconnected from ventilator, extubated and then sent to the morgue after loss of pulse (NB: medical examiner may not authorize potentially traumatic removal of lines and tubes in the case of traumatic cause of injury leading to this death).

Courtesy of Gregory Kapinos, adapted from the 2010 AAN guidelines, Wijdicks EF et al. *Neurology*. 2010;74(23):1911–8, as well as Egea-Guerrero JJ et al. *Neurology*. 2011;76(5):489, Lustbader D et al. *Neurology*. 2011;76(2):119–24 and Frontera JA et al. Neurocrit Care. 2010;12(1):103–10.

CHAPTER 21 ■ PROCEDURES

Maziar Kalani, BS
Melanie G. Hayden Gephart, MD, MAS

CENTRAL LINE

Indication: Central venous pressure (CVP) measurement to assess for fluid status, delivery of parenteral nutrition, delivery of vasopressors or caustic material (chemotherapy, KCl, amiodarone), anticipated extended stay with multiple blood draws and drips, emergent venous access, need to float a Swan-Ganz catheter

Contraindications: Known deep vein thrombosis or aberrant anatomy of vessel, coagulopathy, infection over the insertion site, pneumo- or hemothorax on the contralateral side, uncooperative patient, fracture of ipsilateral ribs or clavicle

Complications: Pneumothorax, hemothorax, chylothorax (each with potential need for a chest tube to be placed), erosion of catheter tip into SVC or RA, catheterization of the subclavian/femoral/carotid artery, dissection of a vessel, tethering of catheter, infection, wire or catheter embolization, arrhythmia, improper catheter location, central venous thrombosis with potential for pulmonary embolus

Informed consent: Advise of need for line and the potential complications; warn of the need to be in Trendelenburg with face covered for an extended period of time

SUBCLAVIAN

Positioning: Trendelenburg (15–30° head down) to prevent air emboli (use caution in high intracranial pressure, congestive heart failure), turn the head to the contralateral side, may put a towel roll between the shoulder blades

Anatomy: Valveless subclavian vein runs parallel and deep to the middle 3rd of the clavicle

- Subclavian artery is superior/posterior to the vein and they are separated by the anterior scalene muscle
- Thoracic duct is on the left side and lymphatic duct on the right
- Right lung dome is lower than the left

Technique:

1. Gather required equipment (triple lumen or cordis central line kit, sterile saline flush, towel) and request nursing to calibrate transducer and set up monitor. Ensure the patient has appropriate analgesia/anxiolytics and nasal cannula for oxygen. Position the patient in Trendelenberg (with a small towel under the shoulder blade to extend the chest, if desired).

2. Prep the primary site using betadine or chlorhexidine and open the central line kit.
3. Put on cap, mask, sterile gown, and gloves. Do a final prep with the prep sticks contained in the central access kit. Drape with a fenestrated sheet covering the face and entire bed. Flush the ports of the central line with sterile saline.
4. Visualize entry point with index finger at sternal notch and thumb at clavicle and junction of the 1st rib (clavicular bend) i.e., 1 cm caudal to the clavicle at 2/3 the distance from the sternoclavicular joint.
5. Infiltrate 1% lidocaine into the subcutaneous tissue with a 25-gauge needle. Repeat with a 22-gauge needle, aspirating prior to injecting, anesthetizing deeper structures including the periosteum of the clavicle.
6. With an 18-gauge needle on a 5-cc syringe, bevel rostral, needle parallel to the clavicle, puncture the skin 1 cm caudal to the clavicle, aiming for the sternal notch, aspirating lightly while advancing the needle under the clavicle. If no venous blood returns, aim 1 cm above the sternal notch.
7. With venous blood return, rotate the bevel caudal, stabilize the needle and remove the syringe, keeping the hub of the needle occluded (to prevent air embolus).
8. Introduce the J wire, with the curl toward the heart until half of the wire remains out or ectopy is observed.
9. Carefully remove the needle without lacerating the wire, maintaining the wire in control at all times.
10. Enlarge the puncture site around the wire slightly with the scalpel, taking care to not cut the wire.
11. Thread the silastic dilator over the wire to dilate the wire track (not the vein) maintaining control of the wire at all times. Remove the dilator while leaving the wire in place.
12. Introduce the wire to the triple lumen catheter (will emerge from the longest hub) to a distance of 15 cm on right, 16 cm on the left. Remove the wire and advance the catheter.
13. Aspirate and then flush each port.
14. Place sutures to either side of the catheter to hold it at the desired length.
15. Obtain STAT chest X-Ray to rule out pneumo/hemothorax, evaluate position of catheter tip.

■ Pearls

If you're having difficulty getting under the clavicle at a parallel angle, start approach further lateral rather than diving under as a steeper angle will result in a pneumothorax

- Avoid multiple attempts as this may lead to a pneumothorax
- Expenence is associated with a decreased complication rate

INTERNAL JUGULAR

Positioning: Trendelenburg (15–30° head down) to prevent air emboli (use caution in high intracranial pressure, congestive heart failure), turn the head to the contralateral side, utilize ultrasound guidance when available

Anatomy: Identify the triangle formed by the clavicle and the heads of the sternocleidomastoid

- Right side is preferred because it is a straight shot into the right atrium
- Carotid is approximated to and medial/deep to the internal jugular

Technique:

1. Prep same as subclavian.
2. Visualize the entry point (the top of the triangle formed by the two heads of the sternocleidomastoid muscle and clavicle) and relationship of internal jugular to carotid artery with the ultrasound.
3. Infiltrate 1% lidocaine into the subcutaneous tissue with a 25-gauge needle. Repeat with a 22-gauge needle, aspirating prior to injecting, anesthetizing deeper structures.
4. Under ultrasound guidance making sure you are lateral to the carotid, insert the 18-gauge needle on a 5-cc syringe through the skin at a 30° angle, aiming toward the ipsilateral nipple, aspirating lightly while advancing the needle.
5. With venous blood return, stabilize the needle and remove the syringe, keeping the hub of the needle occluded (to prevent air embolus).
6. Steps 4–7 same as subclavian.
7. Introduce the wire to the triple lumen catheter (will emerge from the longest hub) to a distance of 14 cm on right, 17 cm on the left. Remove the wire.
8. Continue same as subclavian.

■ Pearls

On ultrasound, the internal jugular is easily compressible whereas the carotid is obviously pulsatile

- Avoid multiple attempts as it increases the risk for pneumothorax or carotid puncture
- After the wire has been placed, confirm the location with ultrasound
- If the patient is very obese and landmarks are not visible, enter three finger breadths lateral from the midline and up from the clavicle
- If you puncture the carotid, withdraw the needle and apply pressure for 10 minutes

FEMORAL

Positioning: Reverse Trendelenburg (15–30° head up) to help with venous filling, utilize ultrasound guidance when available

Anatomy: Locate the femoral artery inferior to the inguinal ligament; femoral vein should be just medial to the artery (remember the mneumonic VAN: vein, artery, nerve heading lateral to medial)

Technique:

1. Prep same as subclavian.
2. Visualize entry point (inferior to the inguinal ligament, medial to the femoral artery) and confirm with ultrasound.

3. Infiltrate 1% lidocaine into the subcutaneous tissue with a 25-gauge needle. Repeat with a 22-gauge needle, aspirating prior to injecting, anesthetizing deeper structures.
4. Under ultrasound guidance, insert the 18-gauge needle on a 5-cc syringe through the skin at a 45° angle 1 cm medial to the femoral pulse and 2 cm inferior to the inguinal ligament, aiming toward the umbilicus, aspirating lightly while advancing the needle.
5. Continue same as subclavian.

▉ Pearls

Even if the pulse is best felt above the level of the inguinal ligament, do not puncture above because this may result in peritoneal perforation or a pelvic hematoma

- If you puncture the femoral artery, withdraw the needle and apply pressure for 10 minutes

LINE CHANGE OVER A WIRE

Indication: Original line in place for an extended period of time, febrile or leukocytosis thought to be caused by central line (controversial—some think requires a new puncture site)

Contraindications (in addition to those to placing the original line): Infected original skin site, original access by cutdown, line placed emergently with questionable sterile technique, coagulopathy

Complications: Less likely but similar to the original line placement

Positioning: Trendelenburg (15–30° head down) to prevent air embolus

Technique:

1. Prep same as subclavian.
2. Remove sutures from original line.
3. Insert wire into the most distal port of the old line and remove, leaving the wire in place.
4. Thread the new line over the wire (if using a triple lumen, wire will come out of the brown colored catheter as it is the most distal port).
5. Aspirate and then flush each port.
6. Place sutures to either side of the catheter to hold it at the desired length Suture and attach line per previous.
7. STAT CXR
   - Consider sending catheter tip for culture if infection considered.

RADIAL ARTERIAL LINE

Indications: Invasive blood pressure monitoring, frequent arterial blood gas samples

Contraindications: Coagulopathy (relative), neurological or arterial compromise with test occlusion of the radial artery (Allen's test)

Complications: Laceration of the artery, hematoma, ischemia, infection

Informed consent: Advise of need for line and the potential complications

Positioning: Supinate the arm and extend the wrist

- Place in a wrist guard to maintain the position throughout the procedure

Technique:

1. Position and prep the wrist with betadine or chlorhexidine.
2. Infiltrate lidocaine with small gauge needle under the dermis for local anesthesia.
3. Put on sterile gloves.
4. Palpate the radial artery.
5. At a 30–45° angle, place arterial line needle ("arrow") into radial artery, attempting distal then proceeding proximal if initially unsuccessful.
6. With a flash of blood into the arterial line, advance the wire into radial artery.
7. Advance soft line catheter and remove wire while occluding the radial artery more proximally. Attach to prepped monitoring line.

■ **Pearls**

Always open at least two arrows in case you miss on the first try; you can reattempt without having to reglove.

- If you initially had good blood return, but then upon inserting the soft catheter there is no blood return, try slowly removing the catheter while carefully reinserting the wire into the artery
- Don't force the wire or catheter in; if the artery spasms down, just withdraw the wire slightly and readvance otherwise you may create a false tract

SPINAL CSF ACCESS

Contraindications: Coagulopathy, low lying cord, thrombocytopenia, coagulopathy, intracranial hypotension (subdural hematomas), infection over the area of the puncture site, increased intracranial pressure from mass lesion or noncommunicating hydrocephalus (risk of post-LP herniation), uncooperative patient

Complications: Pain, CSF leak requiring blood patch, headache, paralysis, nerve root injury, infection, hemorrhage leading to nere root compression and requiring surgical evacuation, herniation if attempted with elevated ICP and an intracranial mass lesion, subdural from intracranial hypotension, retained catheter (LD)

Informed consent: Advise of need for procedure and the potential complications

Positioning: Left lateral decubitus position with neck in full flexion and knees and hips bent (can measure opening pressure)

- If unable to gain access may sit patient up with knees to chest and neck in full flexion

Anatomy: Goal should be to access the L3/4 or 4/5 intraspinous space

- Spinal cord in most patients terminates at L1
- Ligamentum flavum provides the resistance felt prior to entry of the dura
- Flexing the patient maximally will result in splaying of the spinous process and allowing for easier access to the interspinous space

- Posterior superior iliac crest will designate L3/4
- Can also follow the sacral promontory superior to find L5/S1

LUMBAR PUNCTURE (LP)

Indications: To collect CSF for evaluation of infection, immunologic disorders, cytology (oncology), subarachnoid hemorrhage

- To measure ICP (e.g., infection, communicating hydrocephalus, normal pressure hydrocephalus, benign intracranial hypertension)
- Injection of contrast dye for myelogram, intrathecal antibiotics, or chemotherapeutics
- To relieve pressure/fluid in communicating or normal pressure hydro-cephalus, pseudotumor cerebri

Technique:

1. Identify anatomic landmarks to determine the L4/L5 interspinous space and midline.
2. Open a lumbar puncture kit. Prep area including space above. Put on ster-ile gloves and drape the area.
3. Infiltrate lidocaine with a 25-gauge needle under the dermis for local anes-thesia. Repeat with a larger 20-gauge needle to anesthetize the deeper structures.
4. If opening pressure is required, prepare the manometer and attach to the three-way stopcock.
5. Insert the spinal needle with stylet in place, bevel up, between the spinous processes. One may feel a "give" upon penetrating the ligamentum flavum and entering the dura.
6. Remove the stylet from the spinal needle and attach to the three-way stop-cock and manometer to measure opening and closing pressure.
7. Collect CSF.
8. Measure closing pressure.
9. Reinsert the stylet and withdraw the needle while placing pressure on the puncture site.

Lab tests: Send tubes #1 and #4 for cell count and differential, protein, and glucose; send #2 for gram stain and cultures, #3 for cytology

■ Pearls

Unless contraindicated, take off the full 20 cc of fluid because labs are fre-quently added on, and cytology requires a minimum of 10 cc

- Always have one extra vial of lidocaine available and an extra syringe ready
- If the patient is lying on his or her side and you are not sure that you are directly on midline, ask the patient if he or she feels the needle on one side or the other; this will help direct you
- Angle the needle slightly rostral to be parallel with the spinous process you are slipping between

LUMBAR DRAIN

Indications:

- Frequent CSF collection
- Injection of intrathecal medications including antibiotics, chemotherapeutics, antispasmodics (e.g., baclofen)
- CSF drainage for decreased intraoperative brain retraction (for ruptured aneurysms, skull base surgery), pituitary surgery, to heal CSF leak

Technique:

1. Prep same as lumbar puncture.
2. Prepare the lumbar drain catheter by threading the wire into the drain.
3. Insert the 14-gauge Tuohy needle with stylet in place, bevel up, between the spinous processes. One may feel a "give" upon penetrating the ligamentum flavum and entering the dura.
4. Angle the spinal needle rostral (bevel faces cervical) and remove the stylet.
5. Thread the lumbar drain into 40 cm.
6. Attach the LD connector and three-way stopcock, placing a suture where the drain connects in order to secure it. Stitch the drain to the skin and curl under a sterile 2x2 gauze and dressing. Tape the perimeter and secure the drain to the patient's side.

■ Pearls

Same as lumbar puncture, but includes

- When removing the lumbar drain, do not pull when meeting significant resistance; this can result in retained catheter tip; flexing the patient may help in catheter removal
- Take care when removing the Tuohy needle so as to not lacerate the drain
- Be sure to have a sign overhead advising to not adjust height of bed as this may result in advertent overdrainage of CSF

VENTRICULOPERITONEAL SHUNT TAP

Indications: Diagnostic (rule out infection, failure, or for radionucleotide study) or therapeutic (to relieve increased intracranial pressure from a distally occluded shunt)

Contraindications: Coagulopathy (relative), infection over the shunt site

Complications: Infection, shunt malfunction

Positioning: Patient should be sitting in a comfortable position, head turned to allow for sterile evaluation of shunt

Informed consent: Advise of need for procedure and the potential complications

Equipment: Sterile gloves, betadine, alcohol swab, 25- or 23-gauge butterfly needle, 5-cc syringe x(2), sterile gloves and towels, CSF manometer, gauze, small bandage, CSF culture tube (aerobic and anaerobic), razor, three-way stopcock

Technique:
1. Palpate for the valve reservoir.
2. Shave and prep directly over valve.
3. Penetrate the skin and shunt reservoir with the 25-gauge butterfly needle at a 90° angle (perpendicular to the shunt valve). Attach to manometer and three-way stopcock to the butterfly tubing to evaluate ICP (may not be accurate in setting of proximal obstruction). Fill manometer with sterile saline to evaluate distal runoff.
4. Remove stopcock and attach 5-cc syringe to the butterfly syringe to carefully aspirate. If CSF flows without resistance, the proximal portion is likely patent.
5. Obtain CSF for gram stain, culture, glucose, protein, and cell count with differential.

VENTRICULOSTOMY (EXTERNAL VENTRICULAR DRAIN)

Indications: Measurement of intracranial pressure with therapeutic drainage of CSF

Contraindications: Coagulopathy, thrombocytopenia, slit ventricles, infection over incision site

Complications: Intracraanial hemorrhage (subdural, epidural, intraventricular, intraparenchymal), infection, upward herniation (posterior fossa lesion), retained catheter, misplaced catheter leading to paralysis, death

Informed consent: Advise of need for procedure and the potential complications

- Many times is done emergently or patient has altered mental status so consent must be a two physician consent and/or obtained from family if available

Positioning: Supine with towel roll under shoulders to slightly extend the neck, head of bed elevated at 30°

- Place marker (e.g., EKG lead) at patient's glabella

Equipment: Intracranial access kit, sterile towels (three), three-way stopcock, MRI extension tubing, EVD trauma catheter, 3–0 Ethilon sutures on a curved needle (3), sterile gloves/gown, hat, mask

Anatomy: Right side (nondominant) generally preferred unless contraindicated in some way

- Place burr hole 1–2 cm anterior to coronal suture
- Goal is to enter the lateral ventricle with the tip at the beginning of the 3rd ventricle (foramen of Monro)
- Avoid the sagittal sinus by staying 3 cm off of midline

Technique:
1. Review head CT. Adjust entry and trajectory based upon intracranial pathology (e.g., shift) and future operative incision site.

2. Position patient. Ensure patient has nasal canula for O_2 and adequate analgesia/anxiolytic.
3. Shave right scalp past midline and coronal suture.
4. Mark entry point (Kocher's point) at midpupillary line and 2 cm anterior to coronal suture or 10–11 cm from nasion/glabella and 3–4 cm from midline. Also mark out a coronal line from the external auditory meatus to the entry point and a line to the ipsilateral medial epicanthus.
5. Open intracranial access kit and place all equipment on field in a sterile fashion.
6. Prep patient. Put on gown and glove. Drape patient
7. Confirm again anatomic landmarks. Remeasure and redraw lines and confirm entry point.
8. Inject local anesthetic, including periosteum.
9. Incise skin 2–3 cm in the sagittal direction. Elevate the periosteum.
10. Request assistance to hold head still in midline position during drilling. Drill skull hole in the trajectory of the EVD placement (toward ipsilateral medial epicanthus, perpendicular to the skull). Irrigate bone particulates with 18-gauge needle and saline.
11. Puncture dura with large-bore needle.
12. Advance EVD catheter with stylet in place, perpendicular to the skull, aiming toward ipsilateral medial epicanthus, to distance of 5 cm at the outer skull table.
13. Remove stylet and with good CSF flow, advance the catheter without the stylet to 6 cm at the outer skull table.
14. Attach the distal catheter to tunneling sharp while always maintaining control of the proximal catheter at the skull edge with the smooth forceps.
15. Tunnel the catheter in a medial posterior direction at least 2 cm from the burr hole site.
16. Pull the catheter through the tunneled hole, maintaining proximal control of the catheter and ensuring it does not kink, advance, or get pulled out.
17. Cut the distal catheter end and carefully discard the sharp tunneler. Ensure CSF continues to flow freely.
18. Attach the distal catheter end to the tapered connector in the trauma EVD kit with the cap in place. Secure with a tie.
19. Secure the catheter with a suture at the exit site. Close the burr hole skin incision with a running stitch. Stitch the catheter (securely, but nonocclusively) two more times to the scalp.
20. Attach the distal catheter to the three-way stopcock and attach to the MRI tubing. Screw the tubing into the EVD CSF collection bag.
21. Adjust EVD bag height to desired level.
22. Order ceftriaxone for infection prophylaxis and continue for duration of drainage.

◾ Pearls

Do not insert the catheter past 6 cm at the skull, because this is unlikely to result in placement within the lateral ventricle (severe injury or death may result). Generally requires antibiotic prophylaxis with ceftriaxone.

INTRAPARENCHYMAL ICP MEASUREMENT (CAMINO)

Positioning, anatomy, consent, contraindications are the same as for EVD placement

Indications: Measurement of intracranial pressure e.g., in trauma patients with intracranial pathology, with GCS less than 8, or global ischemia (e.g., cardiac arrest)

Complications: Bleeding (subdural, epidural, intraparenchymal), infection

Equipment: Intracranial access kit, sterile towels (3), intracranial pressure measuring device, sterile gloves/gown, hat, mask

Technique:

1. Review head CT. Adjust side based upon intracranial pathology and possible need for conversion to EVD.
2. Step 2–9 the same as for EVD placement.
3. Ensure you have attached the drill bit that comes with the intracranial pressure measuring device (bolt or Camino) or else the hole drilled will be too large for the bolt screw.
4. Steps 11, 12 same as for EVD.
5. Screw bolt into the skull, ensuring you do not advance past the inner table
6. Hand the transducer end of the filament to your assistant and zero the transducer.
7. Loosen the cap on the bolt and slowly advance until a good wave form is read.
8. Tighten the bolt cap around the transducer and snap the plastic clear sheath over the bolt.
9. Place a 4x4 gauze around the base of the bolt. Secure this with pink tape

■ Pearls

If ICP reads inappropriately high, without a good waveform, the transducer may be tented on the dura. Reposition generally requires antibiotic prophylaxis with ceftriaxone

REFERENCES

CHAPTER 1

1. Adams H, Adams R, Del Zoppo G, et al. Guidelines for the early management of patients with ischemic stroke: 2005 guidelines update a scientific statement from the Stroke Council of the American Heart Association/ American Stroke Association. *Stroke*, 2005.
2. Brazis P, Masdeu J, Biller J. *Localization in Clinical Neurology*. 5thed. Philadelphia: Lippincott Williams & Wilkins, 2007.
3. Ellison DW, Love S. *Neuropathology*. 1st ed. St. Louis: Mosby, 1998.
4. Rosamond W, Flegal K, Friday G, et al. Heart disease and stroke statistics–2007 update: a report from the American Heart Association Statistics Committee and Stroke Statistics Subcommittee. *Circulation* 2007;115:e69–171.
5. Greenberg. *Handbook of Neurosurgery*.6th ed. New York: Thieme, 2006.
6. Masuhr F, Mehraein S, Einhaupl K. Cerebral venous and sinus thrombosis. *J Neurol* 2004;251:11–23.
7. Ellis RJ, Olichney JM, Thal LJ, et al. Cerebral amyloid angiopathy in the brains of patients with Alzheimer's disease: the CERAD experience, Part XV. *Neurology* 1996;46:1592–6.
8. Greenberg SM. Cerebral amyloid angiopathy: prospects for clinical diagnosis and treatment. *Neurology* 1998;51:690–4.
9. Greenberg SM, Finklestein SP, Schaefer PW. Petechial hemorrhages accompanying lobar hemorrhage: detection by gradient-echo MRI. *Neurology* 1996;46:1751–4.
10. Vinters HV, Gilbert JJ. Cerebral amyloid angiopathy: incidence and complications in the aging brain. II. The distribution of amyloid vascular changes. *Stroke* 1983;14:924–8.
11. Stroke Syndromes [Washington University in St. Louis School of Medicine], 2007. Available at: http://www.strokecenter.org/prof/syndromes/

CHAPTER 2

1. AbouKhaled KJ, Hirsch LJ. Advances in the management of seizures and statusepilepticus in critically ill patients. *Crit Care Clin* 2006;22:637–59; abstract viii.
2. Claassen J, Hirsch LJ, Emerson RG, et al. Treatment of refractory status epilepticus with pentobarbital, propofol, or midazolam: a systematic review. *Epilepsia* 2002;43:146–53.

3. Gastaut H. Classification of status epilepticus. *AdvNeurol* 1983;34: 15–35.
4. Glauser T, Ben-Menachem E, Bourgeois B, et al. ILAE treatment guidelines: evidence-based analysis of antiepileptic drug efficacy and effectiveness as initial monotherapy for epileptic seizures and syndromes. *Epilepsia* 2006;47:1094–120.
5. Hirsch LJ, Claassen J. The current state of treatment of status epilepticus. *CurrNeurolNeurosci Rep* 2002;2:345–56.
6. Kandel E, Schwartz J, Jessel T. *Principles of Neural Science.* 4th ed. New York: McGraw-Hill, 2000.
7. Merrit, LP R. *Merrit's Neurology.* 10th ed. Philadelphia: Lippincott Williams and Wilkins,2000.
8. Mirski MA, Varelas PN. Seizures and status epilepticus in the critically ill. *Crit Care Clin* 2008;24:115–47, ix.
9. Moore S, Psarros T. *The Definitive Neurological Surgery Board Review.* First ed: Blackwell Publishing, 2005.
10. Rossetti AO. Which anesthetic should be used in the treatment of refractory statusepilepticus? *Epilepsia* 2007;48Suppl 8:52–5.
11. Selvitelli M, Drislane FW. Recent developments in the diagnosis and treatment of status epilepticus. *CurrNeurolNeurosci Rep* 2007;7:529–35.
12. Treiman DM. Treatment of convulsive status epilepticus. *Int Rev Neurobiol* 2007;81:273–85.

CHAPTER 3

1. Rengachary D. *Neurology Survival Guide.* 1st ed. Philadelphia, PA: Lippincott Williams and Wilkins, 2004.
2. Waxman S. *Clinical Neuroanatomy.* 25th ed. New York, NY: Lange Medical Books/McGraw Hill, 2003.

CHAPTER 4

1. Adams R, Victor M, Ropper A. *Principles of Neurology.* New York, NY: McGraw-Hill, Health Professions Division, 1997.
2. Greenberg MS. *Handbook of Neurosurgery. 5th ed.*New York, NY: Thieme, 2001.
3. Massey EW, Schoenberg B. Foster Kennedy syndrome. *Arch Neurol* 1984;41:658–659.
4. Schatz NJ, Smith JL. Non-tumor causes of the Foster Kennedy syndrome. *J Neurosurg* 1967;27:37–44.
5. Tijssen CC, van Gisbergen JA, Schulte BP. Conjugate eye deviation: side, site, and size of the hemispheric lesion. *Neurology* 1991;41:846–850.
6. Moffi e D, Ongerboer de Visser BW, Stefanko SZ. Parinaud's syndrome. *J NeurolSci* 1983;58:175–183.
7. Wall M, Wray SH. The one-and-a-half syndrome—a unilateral disorder of thepontinetegmentum: a study of 20 cases and review of the literature. *Neurology* 1983;33:971–980.

8. La Mantia L, Curone M, Rapoport AM, et al. Tolosa-Hunt syndrome: critical literature review based on IHS 2004 criteria. *Cephalalgia* 2006;26:772–781.

9. Purves D, Augustine G, Fitzpatrick D, et al. *Neuroscience. 4th ed.* Sunderland, MA: Sinauer *Associates*, 2008.

10. NIDCD Information Clearinghouse. Méniére's disease.Bethesda, MD: *NIH Publication*, 2001.

11. Gardner G, Robertson JH. Hearing preservation in unilateral acoustic neuroma surgery. *Ann OtolRhinolLaryngol* 1988;97:55–66.

CHAPTER 5

1. Worldwide Education and Awareness for Movement Disorders. http://wemove.org/, Last updated Mar 23, 2010. Date accessed April 26, 2010.

2. Greenberg. *Handbook of Neurosurgery.*5th ed. New York, NY: Thieme, 2001.

3. Moore S, Psarros T. *The Definitive Neurological Surgery Board Review.* 3rd ed. Philadelphia, PA: Lippincott Williams & Wilkins, 2005.

4. Patten J. *Neurological Differential diagnosis.* 2nd ed. Philadelphia, PA: Springer, 1996.

5. Rowland L, Merritt H. *Merritt's Neurology.* 10th ed. Philadelphia, PA: Lippincott Williams & Wilkin, 2000.

6. Pahwa R, Lyons K. Essential tremor: differential diagnosis and current therapy. *Am J Med* 2003;115:134–142.

7. Coenen VA, Allert N, MaÄNdler B. A role of diffusion tensor imaging fi ber tracking in deep brain stimulation surgery: DBS of the dentato-rubrothalamic tract (drt) for the treatment of therapy-refractory tremor. *Acta Neurochir*(Wien) 2011 Aug; 153(8): 1579–85; discussion 1585.

8. Singer C, Velickovic M. Cervical dystonia: etiology and pathophysiology. *NeurolClin* 2008;26:9–22.

9. Betarbet R, Sherer TB, Di Monte DA, et al. Mechanistic approaches to Parkinson's disease pathogenesis.*Brain Pathol* 2002;12:499–510.

10. Lewitt P. Levodopa for the treatment of Parkinson's disease. *N Engl J Med* 2008;359:2468–2476.

11. Sherer TB, Betarbet R, Greenamyre JT. Environment, mitochondria, and Parkinson's disease.*Neuroscientist* 2002;8:192–197.

CHAPTER 6

1. Mathisen GE, Johnson JP. Brain abscess. *Clin Infect Dis* 1997;25:763–779; quiz 80–81.

2. Koppel B. Bacterial, Fungal, & Parasitic Infections of the Nervous System. In: Brust J, ed. *Current Diagnosis and Treatment in Neurology.* New York, NY: McGraw-Hill Professional, 2006.

3. Parsonnet J. Osteomyelitis. In: Fauci A, Braunwald E, Kasper D, et al., eds. Harrison's Principles of Internal Medicine. 17th ed. New York, NY: McGraw-Hill Professional, 2009: 2754.

4. Tunkel AR, Hartman BJ, Kaplan SL, et al. Practice guidelines for the management of bacterial meningitis. *Clin Infect Dis* 2004;39:1267–1284.
5. Castillo M. *Neuroradiology Companion: Methods, Guidelines, and Imaging Fundamentals*. 3rd ed. Philadelphia, PA: Lippincott Williams & Wilkins, 2005.

CHAPTER 7

1. Moore S, Psarros T. The Definitive Neurological Surgery Board Review. *1st ed*. Malden, MA: Blackwell Publishing, 2005.
2. Larsen P, Stensaas S. PediNeuroLogic Exam. University of Nebraska, University of Iowa Schools of Medicine. Last updated 2007. URL: *http://library.med.utah.edu/neurologicexam/html/home_exam.html*. Last accessed April, 2010.
3. Rothrock S. Tarascon Pediatric Emergency Medicine.*3rd ed. Lompoc, CA: Tarascon Inc.*, 2007.
4. Merrit, LP R. *Merritt's Neurology*. 10th ed. Philadelphia: Lippincott Williams &Wilkins, 2000.
5. Wilkins R, Rengachargy S. *Neurosurgery. 2nd ed.* New York: McGraw-Hill, 1984.
6. Winn HR. *Youman's Neurological Surgery. 5th ed.* Philadelphia: Elsevier, 2004.
7. Osborn A. *Diagnostic Neuroradiology*. St. Louis, MO: Mosby, 1993.
8. Cohen M. *Craniosynostosis: Diagnosis, Evaluation, and Management. 1st ed.* New York: Raven Press, 1986.
9. Cohen MM Jr., Kreiborg S. An updated pediatric perspective on the Apert syndrome. *Am J Dis Child* 1993;147:989–993.
10. Castillo M. *Neuroradiology Companion: Methods, Guidelines, and Imaging Fundamentals*. 3rd ed. Philadelphia, PA: Lippincott Williams & Wilkins, 2005.
11. Meine JG, Schwartz RA, Janniger CK. Klippel-Trenaunay-Weber syndrome. *Cutis* 1997;60:127–132.
12. Gailloud P, O'Riordan DP, Burger I, et al. Diagnosis and management of vein of galen aneurysmal malformations. *J Perinatol* 2005;25:542–551.
13. Albright A, Adelson P, Pollack I. *Principles and Practice of Pediatric Neurosurgery. 1st ed.* New York, NY: Thieme, 2007.
14. Greenberg MS. *Handbook of Neurosurgery. 6th ed.*New York: Thieme, 2006.

FURTHER READING

Aicardi J. The place of neuronal migration abnormalities in child neurology. *Can J NeurolSci* 1994;21:185–193.
Donkelaar H, Lammens M, Hori A, et al. *Clinical Neuroembryology*. Ann Arbor, Michigan. *Springer*, 2006. Sodicoff M. *Embryology of the CNS. Oxford University Press*, 2004.

CHAPTER 8

1. Castillo M. *Neuroradiology Companion: Methods, Guidelines, and Imaging Fundamentals.* 3rd ed. Philadelphia, PA: Lippincott Williams & Wilkins, 2005.
2. Citow J, Macdonald R, Kraig M, et al. *Comprehensive Neurosurgery Board Review.* New York, NY: Thieme, 2000.
3. Greenberg MS. Handbook of Neurosurgery. *5th ed.* New York, NY: Thieme, 2001.
4. Lindsay K, Bone I, Callander R, et al. *Neurology and Neurosurgery Illustrated. 4th ed.* New York, NY: Churchill Livingstone, 2004.
5. Louis D, Ohgaki H, Wiestler O. *World Health Organization Classification of Tumors of the Central Nervous System.3rd ed.* Albany, NY: WHO Publication Center, 2007.
6. CBTRUS (2010). *CBTRUS Statistical Report: Primary Brain and Central Nervous System Tumors Diagnosed in the United States in 2004–2006.* Source: Central Brain Tumor Registry of the United States, Hinsdale, IL. website: www.cbtrus.org.
7. Krouwer HG, Davis RL, Silver P, et al. Gemistocyticastrocytomas: a reappraisal. *J Neurosurg*1991;74:399–406.
8. Lamont JM, McManamy CS, Pearson AD, et al. Combined histopathological and molecular cytogenetic stratification of medulloblastoma patients. *Clin Cancer Res* 2004;10:5482–5493.
9. Ducatman BS, Scheithauer BW, Piepgras DG, et al. Malignant peripheral nerve sheath tumors. A clinicopathologic study of 120 cases. *Cancer* 1986;57:2006–2021.
10. Bellastella A, Bizzarro A, Coronella C, et al. Lymphocytic hypophysitis: a rare or underestimated disease? *Eur J Endocrinol* 2003;149:363–376.
11. Sharma RR. Hamartoma of the hypothalamus and tuber cinereum: a brief review of the literature. *J Postgrad Med* 1987;33:1–13.
12. Ryan M, Shields G. Congenital midline nasal masses. In Quinn F, Ryan M, eds. Grand Rounds, *University of Texas Medical Branch, Department of Otolaryngology,* 2002. Galveston, TX.

CHAPTER 10

1. Acromegaly [NIH Publication No. 08–3924], http://endocrine.niddk.nih.gov/pubs/acro/acro.htm, Bethesda, MD, 2010.
2. Chrousos G, Fradkin J. *National Institute of Diabetes and Digestive and Kidney Diseases [NIH Publication No 04–3054],* 2004.
3. Kumar, Abbas, Fausto. Robbins and Cotran Pathologic Basis of Disease. *7th ed.* New York: Elsevier-Saunders, 2005.
4. Levy A. Pituitary disease: presentation, diagnosis, and management. *J NeurolNeurosurg Psychiatry* 2004;75Suppl 3:iii47–52.
5. Verbalis JG, Goldsmith SR, Greenberg A, et al. Hyponatremia treatment guidelines 2007: expert panel recommendations. *Am J Med* 2007;120:S1–21.

6. Nicholas JA, Burstein CL, Umberger CJ, et al. Management of adrenocortical insufficiency during surgery. *AMA Arch Surg* 1955;71:737–742.

7. Ten S, New M, Maclaren N. Clinical review 130: Addison's disease 2001. *J ClinEndocrinolMetab* 2001;86:2909–2922.

8. Bartter FC, Schwartz WB. The syndrome of inappropriate secretion of antidiuretic hormone. *Am J Med* 1967;42:790–806.

9. Harrigan MR. Cerebral salt wasting syndrome: a review. *Neurosurgery* 1996;38:152–160.

10. Freda PU, Post KD. Differential diagnosis of sellar masses.*Endocrinol MetabClin North Am* 1999;28:81–117, vi.

11. Gsponer J, De Tribolet N, Deruaz JP, et al. Diagnosis, treatment, and outcome of pituitary tumors and other abnormal intrasellar masses. Retrospective analysis of 353 patients. *Medicine (Baltimore)* 1999;78:236–269.

12. Thorner MO and Melmed S. *Prolactinoma [NIH Publication No 02–3924]*, http://endocrine.niddk.nih.gov/pubs/prolact/prolact.htm, Bethesda, MD, 2002.

CHAPTER 11

1. Osborn *A. Diagnostic Neuroradiology. 1st ed.* St Louis, MO: Mosby-Year Book, Inc., 1994.

2. Osborn A, Blaser S, Salzman K, et al. Diagnostic Imaging: Brain. *1st ed. Salt Lake City, UT: Amirsys, Inc., 2004.*

3. Chin L, Regine W. *Principles and Practice of Stereotactic Radiosurgery.* New York, NY: Springer, 2008.

4. Yuh WT, Mayr-Yuh NA, Koci TM, et al. Metastatic lesions involving the cerebellopontine angle. *AJNR Am J Neuroradiol*1993;14:99–106.

5. Thapar K. *Diagnosis and Management of Pituitary Tumors.* Totowa, NJ: Humana Press, 2001.

6. Rao V, Flanders A, Tom B. *MRI and CT Atlas of Correlative Imaging in Otolaryngology. London, UK:* Taylor & Francis, 1993.

7. Ojiri H, Ujita M, Tada S, et al. Potentially distinctive features of sinonasal inverted papilloma on MR imaging. *AJR Am J Roentgenol* 2000;175:465–468.

8. Meyers S. *MRI of Bone and Soft Tissue Tumors and Tumorlike Lesions.* New York, NY: Thieme, 2008.

9. Bianchi D, Crombleholme T, ME DA. *Fetology: Diagnosis and Management of the Fetal Patient. 1st ed.* New York, NY: McGraw-Hill Professional, 2000.

10. Castillo M. *Neuroradiology Companion: Methods, Guidelines, and Imaging Fundamentals. 3rd ed.* Philadelphia, PA: Lippincott Williams & Wilkins, 2005.

11. Osborn A. *Diagnostic Neuroradiology.* St Louis, MO: Mosby, 1993.

12. Mohr JP, Choi DW, Grotta JC, et al. Stroke. *4th ed.* Philadelphia, PA: Elsevier Health Sciences, 2004.

13. Hesselink J. Fundamentals of MR Spectroscopy. Available at: http://spinwarp.ucsd.edu/NeuroWeb/Text/mrs-TXT.htm, 2010.

14. Sankar T, Assina R, Karis JP, et al. Neurosurgical implications of mannitol accumulation within a meningioma and its peritumoral region demonstrated by magnetic resonance spectroscopy: case report. *J Neurosurg* 2008;108:1010–1013.

CHAPTER 12

1. Benzel EC. *Spine Surgery*. 2nd ed. Philadelphia, PA: Elsevier. 2005.
2. Bradford D, Zdeblick TA. *The Spine: Master Techniques in Orthopaedic Surgery*. 2nd ed: *Lippincott Williams, & Wilkins*, Philadelphia, PA. 2004.
3. Vaccaro AR. Fractures of the Cervical, Thoracic and Lumbar Spine. *New York: Informa Health Care*, 2002.
4. Vaccaro AR, Albert TJ. *Spine Surgery: Tricks of the Trade. 2nd ed.*Thieme, NT, NY, 2003.
5. Vaccaro AR, Betz RR, Zeidman SM. Principles and Practice of Spine Surgery. *St. Louis, MO: Mosby*, 2002.
6. Rispoli D. *Tarascon Pocket Orthopaedica. 2nd ed.* Jones & Bartlett Sudbury, MA. 2005.
7. *AnnSurg*85:839–857, 1927.
8. *Spine*5:117–125, 1980.
9. Chesnut RM. Management of brain and spine injuries. *Crit Care Clin*2004;20:25–55.
10. Greenberg M. *Handbook of Neurosurgery. 5th ed.* :Thieme, 2001.
11. Waters RL, Adkins RH, Yakura JS. Definition of complete spinal cord injury. *Paraplegia* 1991;29:573–581.
12. Simon SR. Orthopedic Basic Science, 2nd ed. Page 354, Rosemont, IL AAOS, 1994
13. Schneider R, Crosby E, Russo R, et al. Traumatic spinal cord syndromes and their management. *ClinNeurosurg*1972;20:424–492.
14. Bracken MB, Shepard MJ, Collins WF, et al. A randomized, controlled trial of methylprednisolone or naloxone in the treatment of acute spinal-cord injury. Results of the Second National Acute Spinal Cord Injury Study. *N Engl J Med* 1990;322:1405–1411.
15. Bracken MB, Shepard MJ, Collins WF Jr., et al. Methylprednisolone or naloxone treatment after acute spinal cord injury: 1-year follow-up data. Results of the second National Acute Spinal Cord Injury Study. *J Neurosurg* 1992;76:23–31.
16. Bracken MB, Shepard MJ, Holford TR, et al. Administration of methylprednisolone for 24 or 48 hours or tirilazadmesylate for 48 hours in the treatment of acute spinal cord injury. Results of the Third National Acute Spinal Cord Injury Randomized Controlled Trial. National Acute Spinal Cord Injury Study. *JAMA* 1997;277:1597–1604.
17. Greenberg M. *Handbook for Neurosurgery. 6th ed.* New York: Thieme, 2006.
18. Moore S, Psarros T. *The Definitive Neurological Surgery Board Review. 1st ed.*: Blackwell Publishing, Malden, MA. 2005.

19. Schwartz E, Flanders A. *Spinal Trauma: Imaging, Diagnosis, and Management. 1st ed.:* Lippincott Williams & Wilkins, Philadelphia, PA. 2006.

20. *Pediatrics* 2001;108:e20

21. *Spine 8.*

22. Anderson LD, D'Alonzo RT. Fractures of the odontoid process of the axis. *J Bone Joint Surg Am* 1974;56:1663–1674.

23. Kenter K, Worley G, Griffin T, et al. Pediatric traumatic atlanto-occipital dislocation: five cases and a review. *J PediatrOrthop*2001;21:585–589.

24. Riew KD, Hilibrand AS, Palumbo MA, et al. Diagnosing basilar invagination in the rheumatoid patient. The reliability of radiographic criteria. *J BoneJoint Surg Am* 2001;83-A:194–200.

25. Nassr A, Lee JY, Dvorak MF, et al. Variations in surgical treatment of cervical facet dislocations. *Spine* 2008;33:E188–193.

26. Ordonez BJ, Benzel EC, Naderi S, et al. Cervical facet dislocation: techniques for ventral reduction and stabilization. *J Neurosurg* 2000;92:18–23.

27. Pal GP, Routal RV, Saggu SK. The orientation of the articular facets of the zygapophyseal joints at the cervical and upper thoracic region. *J Anat* 2001;198:431–441.

28. Anderson/Montesano

29. Levine/Edwards

30. Anderson/D'Almso

31. Bono CM. The halo fixator. *J Am AcadOrthopSurg*2007;15:728–737.

32. Herkowitz H. *The Cervical Spine Surgery Atlas. 2nd ed.* Philadelphia: PA, Lippincott Williams & Wilkins, 2003.

33. Choo JH, Liu WY, Kumar VP. Complications from the Gardner-Wells tongs. *Injury* 1996;27:512–513.

34. Netterville JL, Koriwchak MJ, Winkle M, et al. Vocal fold paralysis following the anterior approach to the cervical spine. *Ann OtolRhinolLaryngol*1996; 105:85–91.

35. Kopelson G, Linggood RM, Kleinman GM, et al. Management of intramedullary spinal cord tumors. *Radiology* 1980;135:473–479.

36. Beltran J, Simon D, Levy M. Aneurysmal bone cysts: MR imaging at 1.5 T. *Radiology* 1986;158:689–690.

37. Dahnert W. *Bone and Soft-Tissue Disorders. 2nd ed.* Philadelphia: PA, Lippincott, Williams and Wilkins, 1993.

38. Mishra R, Kaw R. Foix-Alajouanine syndrome: an uncommon cause of myelopathy from an anatomic variant circulation. *South Med J* 2005;98:567–569.

39. Ellison DW, Love S. Neuropathology. *1st ed.* St. Louis, MO: Mosby, 1998.

40. Fielding JW, Hensinger RN, Hawkins RJ. OsOdontoideum. *J Bone Joint Surg Am* 1980;62:376–383.

41. McBride WZ. Klippel-Feil syndrome. *Am Fam Physician* 1992;45:633–635.

42. Thomsen MN, Schneider U, Weber M, et al. Scoliosis and congenital anomalies associated withKlippel-Feil syndrome types I–III. *Spine* 1997;22:396–401.

43. Rothrock S. T*arascon Pediatric Emergency Medicine 1st ed.* Lompoc: Tarascon Inc., 2007.
44. Lustrin ES, Karakas SP, Ortiz AO, et al. Pediatric cervical spine: normal anatomy, variants, and trauma. *Radiographics*2003;23:539–560.
47. Kriss VM, Kriss TC. SCIWORA (spinal cord injury without radiographic abnormality) in infants and children. *ClinPediatr (Phila)* 1996;35:119–124.
48. Pang D, Pollack IF. Spinal cord injury without radiographic abnormality in children—the SCIWORA syndrome. *J Trauma* 1989;29:654–664.
49. Bosch PP, Vogt MT, Ward WT. Pediatric spinal cord injury without radiographic abnormality (SCIWORA): the absence of occult instability and lack of indication for bracing. *Spine* 2002;27: 2788–2800.

CHAPTER 13

1. Greenberg, MS. *Handbook of Neurosurgery.6th ed.* New York: Thieme, 2006.
2. Wirth F. Surgical treatment of incidental intracranial aneurysms. *Clin Neurosurg*1986;33:125–135.
3. Fisher CM, Kistler JP, Davis JM. Relation of cerebral vasospasm to subarachnoid hemorrhage visualized by computerized tomographic scanning. *Neurosurgery* 1980;6:1–9.
4. Claassen J, Bernardini GL, Kreiter K, et al. Effect of cisternal and ventricular blood on risk of delayed cerebral ischemia after subarachnoid hemorrhage: the Fisher scale revisited. *Stroke* 2001;32:2012–2020.
5. Hunt WE, Hess RM. Surgical risk as related to time of intervention in the repair of intracranial aneurysms. *J Neurosurg*1968;28:14–20.
6. Frontera J, Claassen J, Schmidt J, et al. Prediction of symptomatic vasospasm after subarachnoid hemorrhage: the Modified Fisher Scale. *Neurosurgery* 2006;59:21–27.
7. White P, Wardlaw J. Unruptured intracranial aneurysms: prospective data have arrived. *Lancet* 2003;362:90–91.
8. Hartmann A, Mast H, Mohr JP, et al. Morbidity of intracranial hemorrhage in patients with cerebral arteriovenous malformation. *Stroke* 1998;29:931–934.
9. Spetzler RF, Martin NA. A proposed grading system for arteriovenous malformations.*J Neurosurg*1986;65:476–483.
10. Arnautovic K, Krisht A. Transverse-sigmoid sinus duralarteriovenous malformations. *Contemp Neurosurg*;21:1–6.
11. Einhaupl KM, Villringer A, Meister W, et al. Heparin treatment in sinus venous thrombosis. *Lancet* 1991;338:597–600.
12. Sundt TM Jr., Piepgras DG. The surgical approach to arteriovenous malformations of the lateral and sigmoid dural sinuses. *J Neurosurg* 1983;59:32–39.
13. Steiger HJ, Tew JM Jr. Hemorrhage and epilepsy in cryptic cerebrovascular malformations. *Arch Neurol*1984;41:722–724.

14. Wilkins R, Rengachargy S. *Principles of Neurosurgery*. New York: McGraw-Hill,1994.

15. Bousser MG, Chiras J, Bories J, et al. Cerebral venous thrombosis—a review of 38 cases. *Stroke* 1985;16:199–213.

16. Graeb D, Dolman C. Radiological and pathological aspects of duralarteriovenous fistulas. *J Neurosurgery* 1984;15:332–339.

17. Horowitz M, Purdy P, Unwin H, et al. Treatment of dural sinus thrombosis using selective catheterization and urokinase. *Ann Neurol*1995;38:58–67.

18. Caplan LR, Zarins CK, Hemmati M. Spontaneous dissection of the extracranial vertebral arteries. *Stroke* 1985;16:1030–1038.

19. Halbach VV, Higashida RT, Dowd CF, et al. Endovascular treatment of vertebral artery dissections and pseudoaneurysms. *J Neurosurg* 1993;79:183–191.

20. Leys D, Lesoin F, Pruvo JP, et al. Bilateral spontaneous dissection of extracranial vertebral arteries. *J Neurol*1987;234:237–240.

21. Mas JL, Henin D, Bousser MG, et al. Dissecting aneurysm of the vertebral artery and cervical manipulation: a case report with autopsy. *Neurology* 1989;39:512–515.

22. Biller J, Feinberg WM, Castaldo JE, et al. Guidelines for carotid endarterectomy: a statement for healthcare professionals from a special writing group of the Stroke Council, American Heart Association. *Circulation* 1998;97:501–509.

23. Meissner I, Wiebers DO, Whisnant JP, et al. The natural history of asymptomatic carotid artery occlusive lesions. *JAMA* 1987;258:2704–2707.

24. Kashiwagi S, van Loveren HR, Tew JM Jr., et al. Diagnosis and treatment of vascular brain-stem malformations. *J Neurosurg*1990;72:27–34.

25. Chang S, Steinberg G. Surgical management of Moyamoya disease. *ContempNeurosurg*2000;21:1–9.

26. Guzman R, Lee M, Achrol A, et al. Clinical outcome after 450 revascularization procedures for Moyamoya disease. *J Neurosurg*2009; 111:927–935.

27. Ueki K, Meyer FB, Mellinger JF. Moyamoya disease: the disorder and surgical treatment. *Mayo ClinProc*1994;69:749–757.

28. Ellis RJ, Olichney JM, Thal LJ, et al. Cerebral amyloid angiopathy in the brains of patients with Alzheimer's disease: the CERAD experience, Part XV. *Neurology* 1996;46:1592–1596.

29. Greenberg SM. Cerebral amyloid angiopathy: prospects for clinical diagnosis and treatment. *Neurology* 1998;51:690–694.

30. Greenberg SM, Finklestein SP, Schaefer PW. Petechial hemorrhages accompanying lobar hemorrhage: detection by gradient-echo MRI. *Neurology* 1996;46:1751–1754.

31. Moore S, Psarros T. *The Definitive Neurological Surgery Board Review.1st ed.* Philadelphia, PA. Blackwell Publishing, 2005.

32. Osborn A, Blaser S, Salzman K, et al. *Diagnostic Imaging: Brain. 1st ed.* Salt Lake City, UT: Amirsys, Inc., 2004.

CHAPTER 14

1. Alleyne C, Citow J. *Neurosurgery Board Review.2nd ed.* New York, NY: Thieme Medical Publishers, 2005.
2. Castillo M. *Neuroradiology Companion: Methods, Guidelines, and Imaging Fundamentals. 3rd ed.* Philadelphia, PA: Lippincott Williams & Wilkins, 2005.
3. Moore S, Psarros T. *The Definitive Neurological Surgery Board Review. 1st ed.* Philadelphia, PA: Blackwell Publishing, 2005.
4. Osborn A. *Diagnostic Neuroradiology.* St Louis, MO: Mosby, 1993.
5. Wilkins R, Rengachargy S. *Neurosurgery ed.* New York:McGraw-Hill, 1984.
6. McCrory P MW, Johnston K, Dvorak J, Aubry M, Molloy M, Cantu R. Consensus statement on concussion in sport - The 3rd International Conference on concussion in sport, held in Zurich, November 2008. Journal of Clinical Neuroscience. 2009;16:755-63.
7. Rothrock S. *Tarascon Pediatric Emergency Medicine.*Lompoc, ST: Tarascon Inc., 2007.
8. Greenberg, M. *Handbook of Neurosurgery. 5th ed.* New York, NY: Thieme, 2001.

CHAPTER 15

1. Miller M. *Review of Orthopaedics.* Philadelphia, PA: W.B. Saunders, 1992.
2. Netter F. *Atlas of Human Anatomy 1^{st}ed.*: Saunders/Elsevier, 1989.
3. Toothaker TB,Brannagan TH 3rd. Chronic inflammatory demyelinating polyneuropathies: current treatment strategies. *CurrNeurolNeurosci Rep* 2007;7:63–70.
4. Alleyne C, Citow J. *Neurosurgery Board Review. 2nd ed.* New York:Thieme Medical Publishers, 2005.

CHAPTER 16

1. U.S. National Institutes of Health. Deep brain stimulation (DBS) versus best medical therapy (BMT) trial. Available at: http://clinicaltrials.gov/show/NCT00056563. Dept. of Veteran Affairs, Washington, DC.AccessedJanuary 22, 2009.
2. Deep-brain stimulation of the subthalamic nucleus or the pars interna of the globuspallidus in Parkinson's disease. *N Engl J Med* 2001;345:956–963.
3. Anderson VC, Burchiel KJ, Hogarth P, et al. Pallidal versus subthalamic nucleus deep brain stimulation in Parkinson's disease. *Arch Neurol* 2005;62:554–560.
4. Benabid AL, Chabardes S, Mitrofanis J, et al. Deep brain stimulation of thesubthalamic nucleus for the treatment of Parkinson's disease. *Lancet Neurol*2009;8:67–81.

5. Deuschl G, Schade-Brittinger C, Krack P, et al. A randomized trial of deepbrain stimulation for Parkinson's disease. *N Engl J Med* 2006;355:896–908.

6. Kleiner-Fisman G, Herzog J, Fisman DN, et al. Subthalamic nucleus deep brain stimulation: summary and meta-analysis of outcomes. *MovDisord* 2006;21Suppl 14:S290–304.

7. Olanow CW, Watts RL, Koller WC. An algorithm (decision tree) for the management of Parkinson's disease (2001): treatment guidelines. *Neurology* 2001;56:S1–S88.

8. Schupbach WM, Maltete D, Houeto JL, et al. Neurosurgery at an earlier stage of Parkinson disease: a randomized, controlled trial. *Neurology* 2007;68:267–271.

9. Weaver F, Follett K, Hur K, et al. Deep brain stimulation in Parkinson disease: ametaanalysis of patient outcomes. *J Neurosurg* 2005;103:956–967.

10. Weaver FM, Follett K, Stern M, et al. Bilateral deep brain stimulation versus best medical therapy for patients with advanced Parkinson's disease: a randomized controlled trial. *JAMA* 2009;301:63–73.

11. Koulousakis A, Kuchta J. Intrathecalantispastic drug application with implantable pumps: results of a 10-year follow-up study. *ActaNeurochir Suppl* 2007;97:181–184.

12. National Institutes of Health. *Chronic pain: hope through research.* 1982. Bethesda, MD: U.S. Dept. of Health and Human Services, Public Health Service, National Institutes of Health (NIH); Washington, D.C.:82–2406.

13. Fields H. *Pain.* New York: McGraw-Hill Information Services Company, 1987.

14. Cox JJ, Reimann F, Nicholas AK, et al. An SCN9A channelopathy causes congenital inability to experience pain. *Nature* 2006;444:894–898.

15. Gerdle B, Bjork J, Henriksson C, et al. Prevalence of current and chronic pain and their influences upon work and healthcare-seeking: a population study. *J Rheumatol* 2004;31:1399–406.

16. Latham J, Davis BD. The socioeconomic impact of chronic pain. *Disabil Rehabil* 1994;16:39–44.

17. Melzack R, Wall PD. Pain mechanisms: a new theory. *Science* 1965;150:971–979.

18. Waxman SG. Neurobiology: a channel sets the gain on pain. *Nature* 2006;444:831–832.

19. Woolf CJ. Pain: moving from symptom control toward mechanism-specific pharmacologic management. *Ann Intern Med* 2004;140:441–451.

20. National Institutes of Health. *Complex regional pain syndrome fact sheet.* 2003. Available at: www.ninds.nih.gov/disorders/reflex_sympathetic_dystrophy/ detail_reflex_sympathetic_dystrophy.htm. Accessed May 2, 2009.

21. Kavuk I, Yavuz A, Cetindere U, et al. Epidemiology of chronic daily headache. *Eur J Med Res* 2003;8:236–240.

22. Greenberg, M.S. *Handbook of Neurosurgery.* 5th ed. New York: Thieme, 2001.

23. National Institute of Nerological Disorders and Stroke. *NINDS occipital neuralgia information.* 2008. Available at: www.ninds.nih.gov/disorders/ occipitalneuralgia/occipitalneuralgia.htm. Bethesda, MD, Accessed May 3, 2009.
24. Bonica J. The Management of Pain. *2nd ed.* Philadelphia: Lea and Febiger, 1990.
25. Koulousakis A, Kuchta J, Bayarassou A, et al. Intrathecal opioids for intractable pain syndromes. *ActaNeurochirSuppl*2007;97:43–48.

CHAPTER 20

1. Churchill WH. Transfusion therapy. In: *Scientific American Medicine.* Federman D (ed.) New York: Scientific American, Inc.; March 2001.
2. Hebert PC *et al.* A multicenter, randomized, controlled clinical trial of transfusion requirements in critical care.*NEJM* 1999; 340:409–17.
3. Wu W-C *et al.* Blood transfusion in elderly patients with acute MI. *NEJM* 2001; 345:1230–1236.
4. TRAPS Group. Leukocyte reduction and UVB irradiation to platelets to prevent allo-immunization and refractoriness to platelet transfusions.*NEJM* 1997; 337:1861–9.
5. Hotchkiss RS, Karl IE. The pathophysiology and treatment of sepsis. N Engl J Med 2003;348:138–50.
6. Winshall J, Lederman R. Tarascon Internal Medicine and Critical Care Pocketbook. 4th ed. Lompoc: Tarascon, Inc, 2007.

INDEX

Note: Italicized page locators indicate illustrations; tables are noted with *t*.

Stay Connected with Tarascon Publishing!

Monthly Dose eNewsletter
—Tarascon's Monthly eNewsletter

Stay up-to-date and subscribe today at: www.tarascon.com

Written specifically with Tarascon customers in mind, the Tarascon Monthly Dose will provide you with new drug information, tips and tricks, updates on our print, mobile and online products as well as some extra topics that are interesting and entertaining.

Sign up to receive the Tarascon Monthly Dose Today! Simply register at www.tarascon.com.

You can also stay up-to-date with Tarascon news, new product releases, and relevant medical news and information on Facebook, Twitter page, and our Blog.

STAY CONNECTED

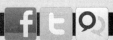

Facebook: www.facebook.com/tarascon
Twitter: @JBL_Medicine
Blog: blogs.jblearning.com/medicine